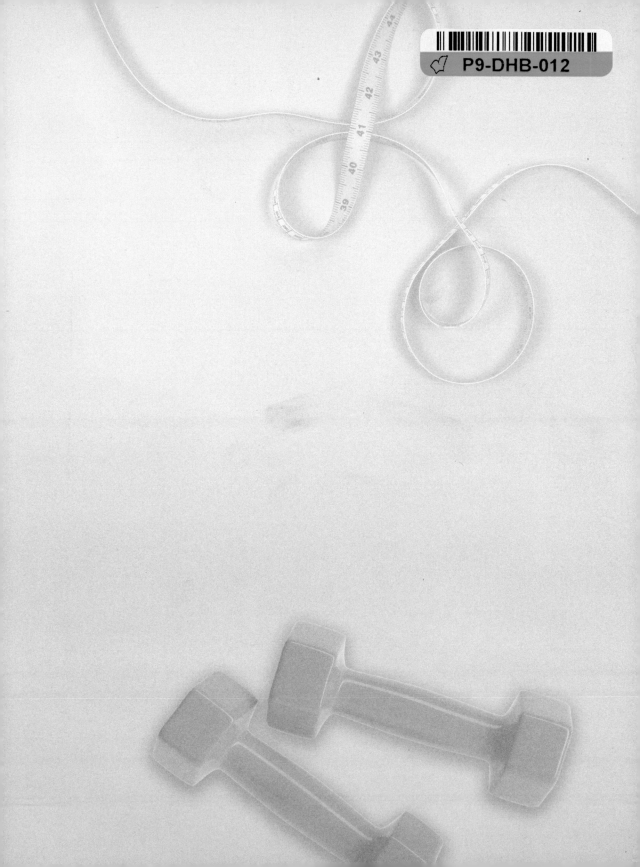

WEIGHT-LOSS HERO

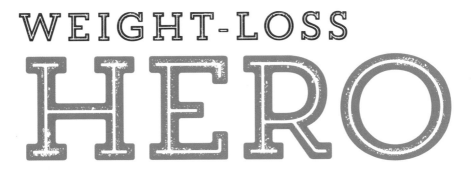

*Transform Your Mind
and Your Body with a Healthy*
KETO LIFESTYLE

CHRISTINE CARTER

ZONDERVAN®

ZONDERVAN

Weight-Loss Hero

Copyright © 2020 by Christine Carter

This title is also available as a Zondervan ebook.

This title is also available as a Zondervan audio book.

Requests for information should be addressed to:

Zondervan, *3900 Sparks Dr. SE, Grand Rapids, Michigan 49546*

ISBN 978-0-3104-5451-9

Art direction: Jennifer Showalter Greenwalt
Interior design: Mallory Collins

Printed in India

20 21 22 23 24 REP 10 9 8 7 6 5 4 3 2 1

I would like to dedicate this book to my brother, Matthew, who taught me to look at the world through a different lens.

. . . .

I'd also like to thank and acknowledge the members of my team and my tribe. Thank you for filling my love cup every day and challenging me to become more.

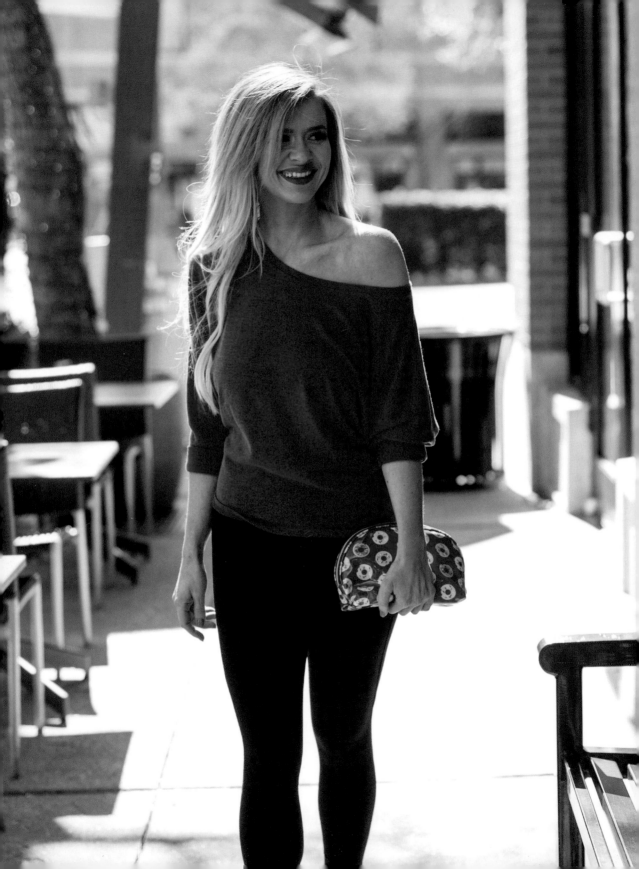

CONTENTS

PART 2: THE KETO DIET

PART 3: THE HEART OF THE WORKOUT

PART 4: SHOPPING LISTS, MEAL PLANS, AND RECIPES

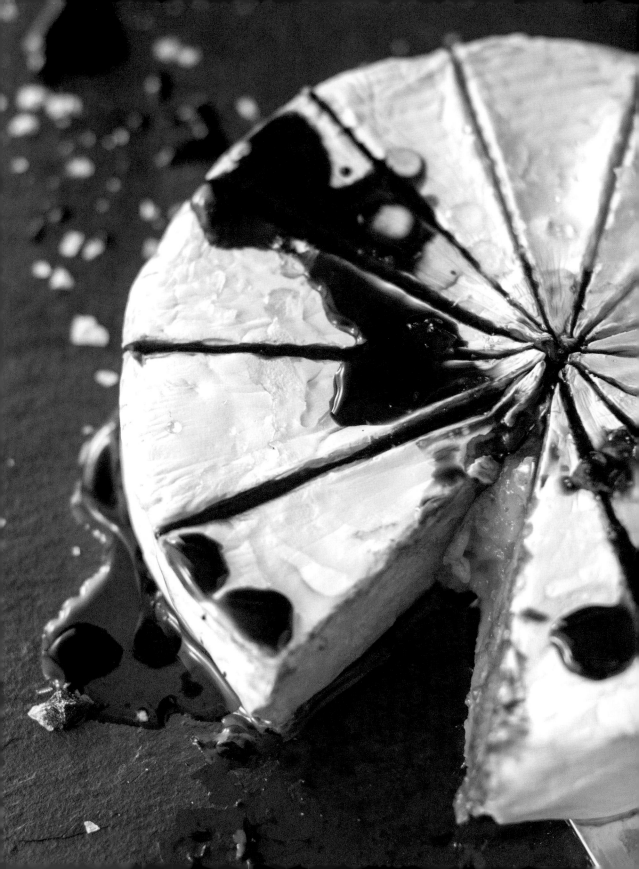

FOREWORD

By Heather Rushin

I am a lover of food and I have made it my mission to share great recipes developed in my home kitchen for the home cook. I love food so much that I have made a life out of recipe development and food photography, so I am fortunate to have turned these passions into a career that is fulfilling and keeps me healthy!

However, I didn't always love food. I went from being a picky child who loved only a handful of foods to a young adult who saw food as the enemy. When I was a teenager, food made me sick with terrible stomach pains. As I got older, food still made me sick—and it also made me fat. For me, no food was good; it was all bad. Just like Christine, I tried just about every diet in existence and they all had the same message: *Food is the enemy. Less is more. Struggle harder for your goal.*

Everything changed when I was introduced to the Paleo lifestyle. I started to see the good in food, but those pesky health issues and the extra weight didn't disappear as I had hoped. Instead it took a chance reading of *Keto Clarity* by Jimmy Moore to provide the final piece of the puzzle for me. And then everything came full circle when Jimmy asked me to co-author the companion cookbook, *Keto Clarity Cookbook*.

Now, without a doubt, I can say I love food and see it as an important tool that brings joy in my daily life.

I am so honored to write the foreword of this amazing resource! Christine is *so* relatable! We all have a diet history and she shows us how to move on from our patterns in a healthy and simple way. She is like a coach, teaching us how to use her book and get the most out of this resource. And I love that Christine recommends that when you read a new idea or exercise in the book to stop reading. Stop and think about the new idea and how it fits into your life, instead of breezing by something new, scary, or different. This is great advice and if you do it, I know you'll get results from this amazing book!

As a professional food blogger and recipe developer, I turn to the recipe section of any book first. The recipes included here are crazy-simple yet flavorful! I am thoroughly impressed and can't wait to try the Breakfast Sausage Balls on page 182 and the Volcano Roll in a Bowl on page 188. Christine says right away, "*Simple recipes are my jam.*" The recipes included in this book are great if you are busy, don't have time for fussy ingredients and cooking methods, or are simply new to cooking.

If there is one important message to get, it's that you are not alone. Christine shares her story so bravely, not to just show how far she has come, but so we can all see another person who has struggled with diet and health. She goes from not wanting to be seen at all, to sharing herself fully with readers. When we see ourselves and our struggles in another person, we can begin to see what is possible for ourselves.

Not only will you discover lots of information and how-tos on changing your lifestyle and eating habits, but you'll also find support and encouragement from someone who has been through the trenches and come out vibrant on the other side. The inspiration and stories along the way make lifestyle change seem real and possible for anyone. Christine instills the most important thing of all through her personal story and journey—hope.

—Heather Rushin

Author of *Keto Clarity Cookbook*

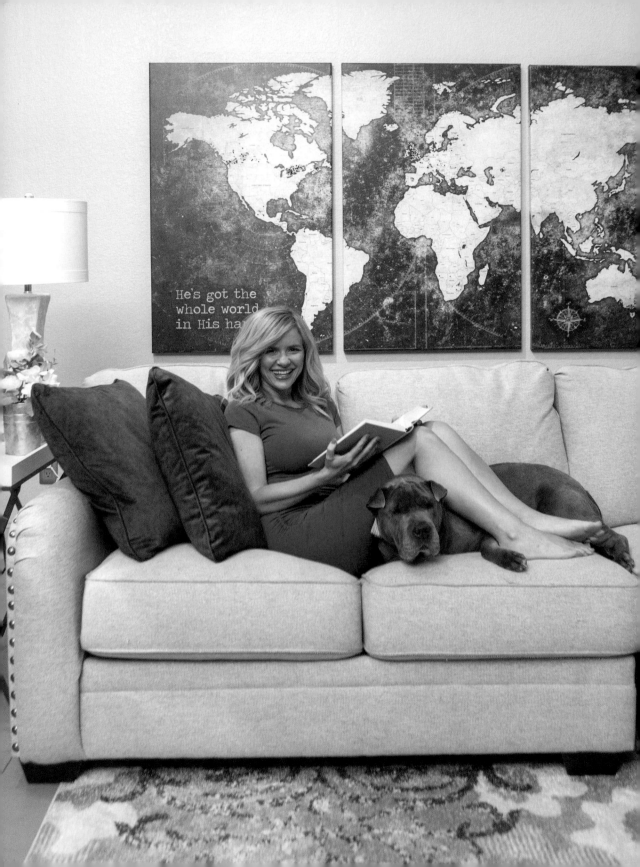

INTRODUCTION

GETTING OFF THE
ROLLER COASTER

I feel like I already know you because I've been you. Sure, our stories and journeys are unique, but we both have faced challenges and found ourselves stuck in the same unhealthy lifestyle. The feeling of hopelessness on this lonely road of being sick-and-tired-of-feeling-sick-and-tired is universal, despite our different circumstances, and I am confident the pages ahead will provide you with some insight and answers for how to take the first steps toward a new life.

My genuine prayer is that as you turn the pages in this book, you find your "Aha!" moment. I ask you to open your heart to the possibility that maybe there is a better life out there waiting for you; you just need to be brave enough to chase after it. My goal is not to be a hero *for* you but to help you discover the hero that already lives inside of you.

To get the best use of this book, I suggest approaching it like a life guide. When you come to a new idea or exercise, set the book down and really think it through, write it out, and put it into motion. Gaining the knowledge to change your life for the better is good, but it is fairly useless if you don't turn that knowledge into action.

My goal is not to be a hero for you but to help you discover the hero that already lives inside of you.

Back in 2014, I felt like I had lost everything . . . *except* the weight. Topping the scales at 297 pounds, I had no direction in life. The harder I tried to lose weight, the harder the process became. I lost my health, my dignity, my confidence, and my happiness. But more important, I lost *myself*. I didn't love myself anymore, and honestly, I didn't even *like* myself.

I tried every diet known to man. I experimented with fad diets, starving myself, and the good ole "lifestyle change"—eat right and exercise—with the hope that somewhere along the way, I would discover the self-control I needed lurking in the shadows of my mind. I even had weight-loss surgery. I just *knew* that surgery would be the fix I had been searching for and would solve all my problems.

Unfortunately, not long after the surgery, I was confronted by the harsh reality that even having a portion of my stomach surgically removed would not save me. I continued to repeat the same patterns—gaining and losing weight—over and over again. I eventually ended up exactly where I had started. I found myself still—even after putting myself through a painful and expensive weight-loss surgery—strapped to the roller-coaster ride I never wanted to be on.

Each time I started a new diet plan, I was all in for a week, maybe even two, until my old habits and routines snuck back up on me. Then I would fall off the crazy ride . . . and fall *hard*. I'd binge eat my way back to where I began, and I always managed to pick up a few extra pounds along the way. I literally dieted my way to 297 pounds.

It's not that the diet plans or fitness plans I tried couldn't have worked; it was my ability to *stick to them* that failed me time and time again. This roller-coaster cycle continued to the point that fear prevented me from even wanting to try again.

Perhaps you can relate on some level. The fear of failing can be absolutely crippling. And the thought of trying again gave me debilitating anxiety that made even breathing feel like a nearly impossible task. The only thing that brought comfort in my life was food, and the idea of taking it away was terrifying.

What if I fail again? What if I can't do it? What if I'm meant to be overweight and live in shame forever?

I LITERALLY DIETED MY WAY TO 297 POUNDS.

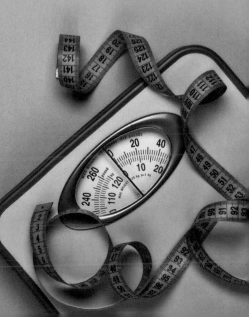

As the number on the scale climbed, so did my depression and anxiety. I was on every prescription drug my doctor could recommend to help me function. I had to take medications for the side effects of other medications. Meds on meds on meds! My entire body hurt, and my mind was a mess. I felt stuck, like there was no way out.

My rock-bottom moment came during a time that should have been fun. I was on my way to a family reunion—one I hadn't attended in years. I felt so ashamed about who I had become, and I didn't want to go. My dad begged and pleaded for me to come, so I pulled myself together enough to get dressed and make the five-hour drive to south Texas.

I remember that morning so vividly. I frantically searched for something to wear that would minimize the excess weight I was carrying. I wanted so badly to blend into the background and hoped no one would notice I was there. I found a solid black T-shirt and a maxi skirt to hide the pounds I believed defined me, and then I reluctantly departed to spend time with people whom I should have been happy to see.

He didn't recognize me because of the 120 pounds I had gained since the last time he had seen me.

When I arrived at the family reunion, I spotted my favorite uncle across the room. I had not seen Uncle Bruce in many years, but to me, it felt as if it were yesterday. He began walking my way to say hello, or so I thought. As Uncle Bruce approached me, he looked me in the eyes, gave a casual nod, said "hi," and kept on walking. *How rude!*

Why didn't he stop to talk to me? Did I do something wrong? Had I offended him somehow? All sorts of anxious and unreasonable thoughts flooded my mind.

I followed him and grabbed him by the shoulder, exclaiming, "Uncle Bruce! It's me! Christine."

He was shocked. He had *no idea* who I was.

I. Was. Devastated.

He didn't recognize me because of the 120 pounds I had gained since the last time he had seen me. I spent the better part of four mortifying minutes trying to explain who I was before my uncle was able to make the connection with the person now standing in front of him.

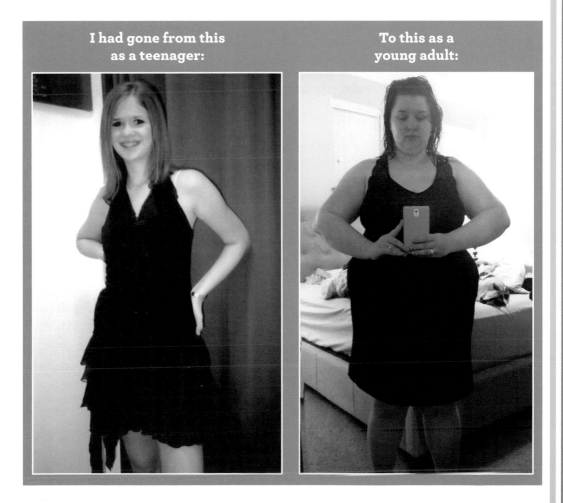

I had gone from this as a teenager:

To this as a young adult:

As you can see, I had literally eaten myself to an unrecognizable state.

As you can see, I had literally eaten myself to an unrecognizable state.

I didn't know much, but when I left, I knew one thing: *I would never feel that way again.*

At my worst moment, I felt completely broken. My self-esteem had been shattered into so many pieces I thought it was beyond repair. I was desperately in need of a total transformation and had no idea where to begin.

When I began my weight-loss journey for the *last* time, hoping to finally get off the emotional roller coaster that had defined my life for far too long, I knew one thing I had to change: if I wanted to fix the outside, I had to fix the inside first. This realization was as exciting as it was terrifying. How does someone fix the inside? Where would I start?

Lucky for me, God had a plan and provided the guidance I needed in the same way I want to guide you. During the journey that lay ahead of me, I slowly began to uncover the warrior within me that had been lost for so long. I embraced a beautiful relationship with God, who was waiting with His arms stretched wide. I finally found *my* breakthrough, and I am here to help you find yours.

. . . .

When I finally got serious, I identified a few things I had to be honest with myself about: I did not like to cook, I did not like to work out, and I liked to eat out. Believe it or not, these were things I didn't have to change. I had a moment of clarity when I realized I didn't have to alter everything about *who I am*. I just had to change *what I did* and *how I thought*. It's less about changing who you are and more about discovering who you were created to be in the first place. This realization allowed me to fully commit to the process. I had to start by examining what was going on inside in order to see the changes on the outside.

Initially I thought I had a weight problem. I believed if I could just lose the weight, all my problems would somehow disappear. However, during this transformative process, I came to realize the weight was not the *cause* of my problems but the *symptom* of something lurking much deeper beneath the surface. If I wanted to see lasting change, something would have to be different this time.

The process I followed to discover those things lurking beneath the surface, preventing me from making real changes and achieving a physical transformation, included a three-pronged approach to weight loss that I will teach you in the pages to come:

1. A total mind-set makeover
2. An effective but simple diet that includes delicious and easy-to-make food
3. Basic and unintimidating workouts

Throughout this journey, I have consistently heard that I am an "overcomer." By definition, an overcomer is someone who has made the best of a conflict. But my story is not that of someone who has overcome. It is a story of a young woman who must decide every day to be brave, bold,

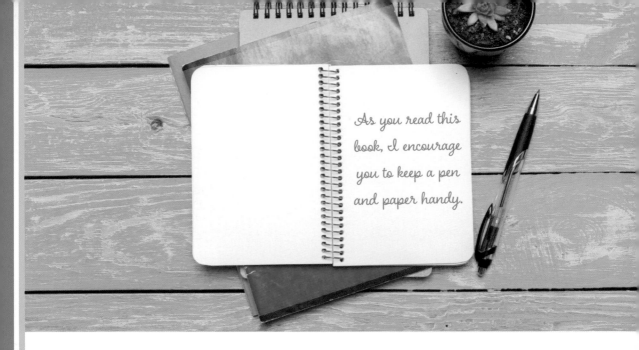

As you read this book, I encourage you to keep a pen and paper handy.

and fearless—even when she can think of every reason not to be. I am not an overcomer, because this journey lasts a lifetime. I will never stop overcoming both new and old challenges in my life.

I quickly realized this process meant slaying the giants that taunted me, overpowering the addictions that crippled me, and challenging the voice in my head that said I wasn't enough. And I am here to help you do the same.

The simple secret to true and lasting change is that it must start in your mind and *burn* through your body. If we don't address what's going on in our heads and our hearts, we will never find the ongoing success we are looking for. You cannot live the life of your dreams while operating in the same mind-set that broke you down.

There are a few mind-set patterns you will need to rewrite. Retraining your brain can take some time, and you *must* learn to be patient and gentle with yourself. You will fail. You will mess this all up—probably more than once. But I am here to help you discover the fighter that lives inside of you who will always come back swinging. Even after taking a punch, you will learn to stand up each and every day and *fight* for the kind of life you want to live—the life you deserve to live.

I fell so much in love with this process of retraining my brain and redefining my own life that I've created a platform to support others on their journey. This passion led me to become a certified personal fitness instructor, with a specialized certification in behavioral change, which is a process I plan to share with you.

As you read this book, keep a pen and paper handy. In the pages ahead, there will be mind-set exercises for you to work through. My request is that you really dive into them, embrace them, and apply them. It is so easy to read something you know would be helpful to incorporate into your life and think, *Oh, I'll do that later*, then move on with your life. While it's true that knowledge is power, it is in the *application* of that knowledge that freedom exists.

You have the power within you to determine your path, so strap on your running shoes and run the beautiful race that is your life. We are on this earth for only a little while, and it's time we make this moment count. Together we will find the seed already planted deep within you, and nurture and love it to become the beautiful flower that is waiting to bloom.

I've had the privilege of helping thousands of women around the world achieve their fitness goals, and now I'm here to help you. Please join me in my mission to make the world a happier and healthier place . . . one pound at a time.

Please join me in my mission to make the world a happier and healthier place . . . one pound at a time.

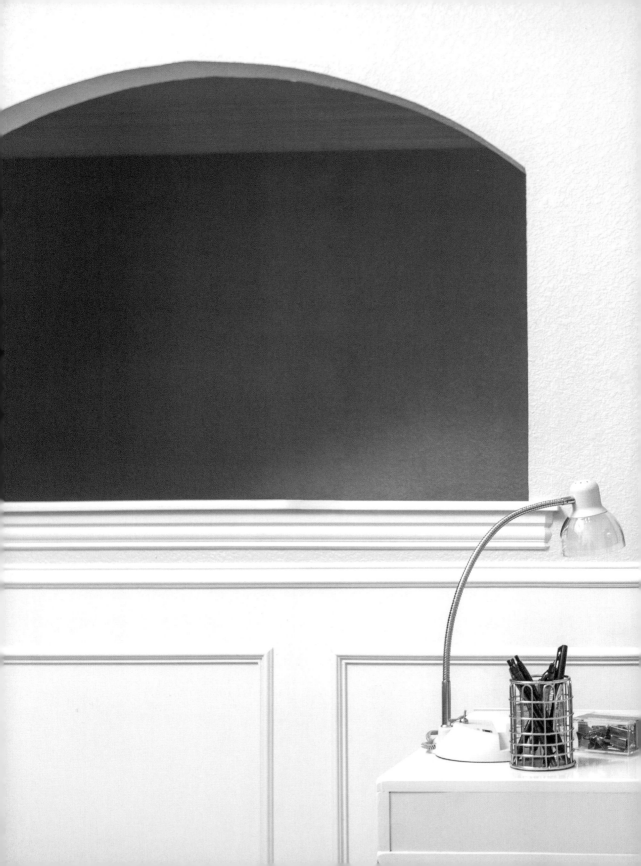

PART 1

YOU ARE WHAT
YOU THINK

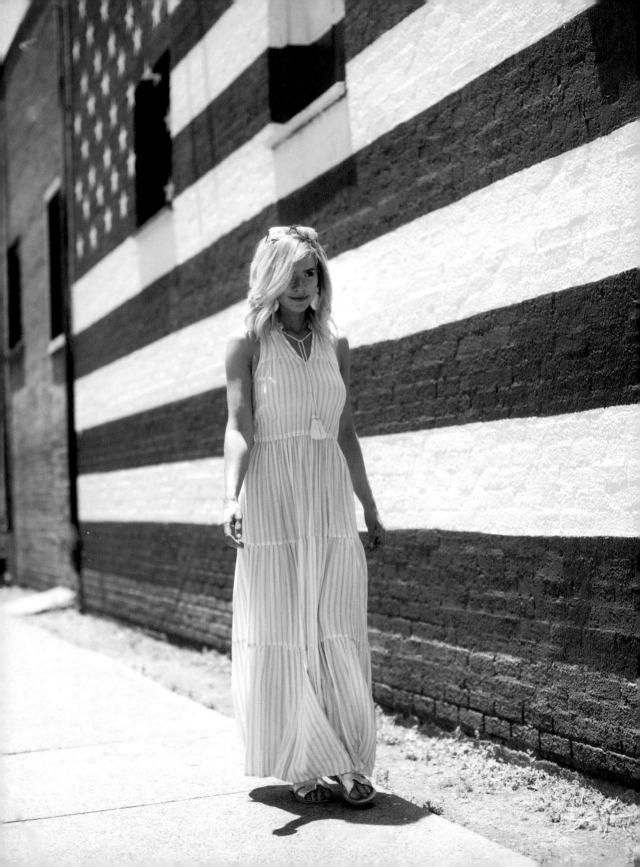

1

WHERE IT ALL BEGAN

I'd like to invite you along my personal journey. Through this journey, and my experience working with thousands of women worldwide, I have found the weight most of us carry is our best effort to put a Band-Aid over a bullet hole. We have spent the majority of our lives being told we aren't supposed to feel feelings, and we are expected to have it all together . . . or at least *look* like we do.

The problem is that we were created to have feelings, and our feelings are *valid*. Most of us have unhealed pain and are seeking something to fill the void of that pain so that maybe we can go one more day without hurting. Food provides us a temporary relief to the feelings we aren't facing, until the very thing pacifying us becomes the thing that's killing us. Killing our mind, killing our body, and killing our spirit.

I didn't want to admit I had problems lurking below my very unhealthy skin surface. I was eating away every undealt-with feeling I had because I didn't want to face the truth.

Food provides us a temporary relief to the feelings we aren't facing, until the very thing pacifying us becomes the thing that's killing us.

Everyone has a story of how they got to their personal breaking point, both physically and mentally. Identifying the catalyst can be a cathartic and productive way to create a new beginning for the rest of your life. Whether you've spent your life battling the genes you were born with or you can identify a momentous or tragic event that changed your path or broke your heart, something significant affected your mind-set and triggered the habits that brought you to where you are today.

It's difficult to pinpoint the exact moment in time when my weight gain began, but there is a specific traumatic event in the fall of 2009 that started a domino effect of change that took me on a ride in the wrong direction. I had gone to a party and afterward was assaulted. I was scared, lost, and felt hopeless. I hid my feelings, and I thought that if I could bury this part of me so deep, maybe not even I could find it.

What I didn't realize was that the emotions I had tried so hard to bury were like an infectious disease deep within my core—a disease that would spread like a wildfire and, eventually, consume me.

The scariest and saddest part of all this is that this phenomenon is not unique to me. During my time as a wellness coach, my eyes have been opened to the prevalence of trauma and abuse in our society and how it affects every aspect of its victims' lives, including long-term, negative effects on health. But there are many other ways in which people's

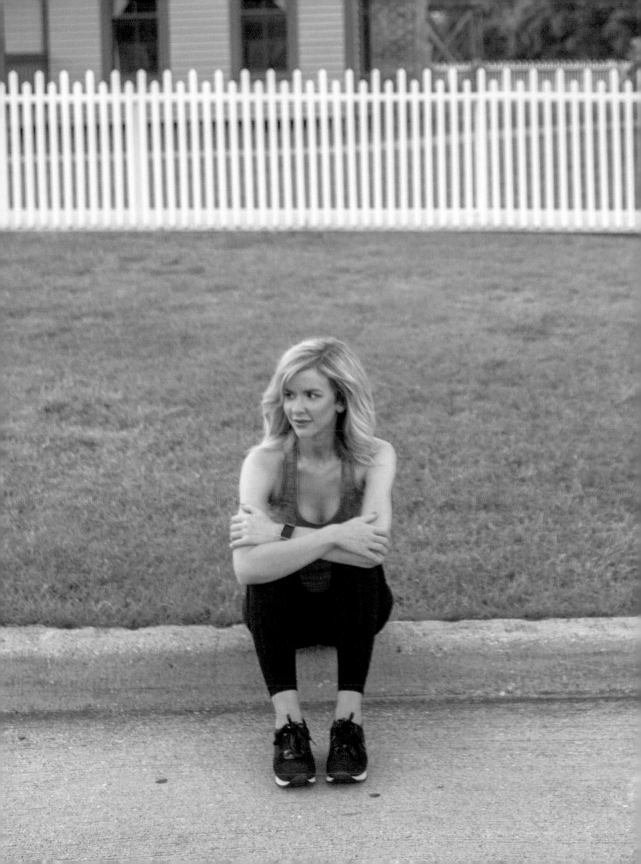

lives have been defined by their pain, leading them to self-destructive behaviors.

Something painful or challenging likely marked a permanent change in your mind-set, or maybe you've felt undeserving of good health for as long as you can remember. For me, it led to developing a binge-eating disorder, where I gained 100 pounds within a short year.

Binge eating disorder is the most common eating disorder in the United States, and according to the National Eating Disorder Association, it is characterized by recurrent episodes of eating large quantities of food (often quickly); a feeling of a loss of control during the binge; and experiencing shame, distress, or guilt.[1] This may or may not sound familiar to you, but it's likely that if you're looking to begin your weight-loss journey, you might recognize the emotions associated with this disorder and have felt ashamed and guilty about your eating habits. These emotions have ultimately impacted your happiness and quality of life as a whole.

I was diagnosed with binge eating disorder when I was twenty-three years old and felt helpless to change. I constantly ate to the point of being sick and experiencing physical pain. As I was eating one meal, I would be thinking about the next. The more I tried to change and restrict myself, the more I felt trapped and the worse my symptoms became.

Whether or not you have suffered from binge eating disorder—diagnosed or not—I promise there is a way out of the unhealthy trap you have created, including steps you can take to make it easier to control your impulses.

I'll talk more in-depth about the evils of sugar in Part 2 of this book, but as you find yourself in the beginning stages of changing your mind-set and taking into account the things you struggle with most, it's crucial to understand that every step you take on this journey to get away from sugar is a step in the right direction. Underlying sugar addiction is a huge culprit (and trigger) for people struggling with weight gain—and binge eaters, specifically.

When I feel I might be slipping into old habits, these are the steps I take to stay on track:

1. I drink a full bottle of water.
2. I eat an on-plan meal until I'm full.
3. I reread my "why" and my vision. (I'll talk more about this in another section.)
4. I promise myself that *if* I do all of these things and then I still want to "cheat" on my diet—or binge—I'm allowed to do so.

UNDERLYING
SUGAR ADDICTION
IS A
HUGE CULPRIT.

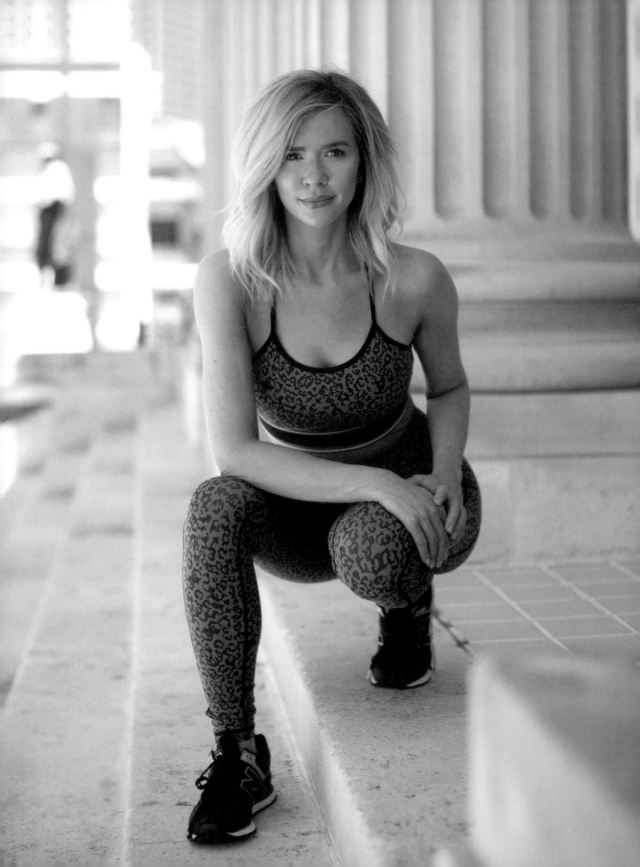

By promising ourselves "not now, but later," we talk ourselves out of the mental restriction that diets can bring. Healthy habits have to be built. It will take time, but the more often you implement them, the stronger you will become.

At this point in my life all I needed was to feel better in the moment. But more than anything, I wanted to feel nothing at all. When thoughts of that life-changing evening flooded my mind, I turned to food as a momentary cure to feel better—even if just for a little while.

I ate carb-laden meals large enough to kill a man. Food made me feel okay. Food made the bad thoughts go away. Food became my savior—the thing I turned to when I didn't know where else to go.

> Food became my savior—the thing I turned to when I didn't know where else to go.

When we consume large amounts of sugar, equally large amounts of dopamine are released into our body. Dopamine has the infamous nickname of "the Molecule for Happiness"[2] because it tricks us into feeling happy. But when that happiness fades, we are back where we started, and we are craving more of it.

I often asked myself, *Why can't I stop eating? Why can't I stop thinking about food?* I thought I was crazy. The more I ate, the more weight I gained. And truthfully, I didn't mind . . . at first. It made me feel safe. The problem, though, was that I was becoming my own abuser. I was the only one responsible for the continued mistreatment I inflicted on myself for many years.

In a matter of a year, I gained one hundred pounds. I ate myself sick. I attempted to use food to heal my broken spirit. Though it made me feel good for a moment, this pattern set me up for a tremendous amount of pain.

I will never feel this way again.

I began going through the motions in my life. I wasn't really living life; life was living me. I most certainly was not *loving* my life. Though deeply wounded, I did continue moving forward. I found a good job, got married, and bought a house, but I still felt so empty inside. Food was my only source of comfort even though it was also tearing me apart.

After my family reunion in June of 2014, I'd had enough. I was completely fed up with my life and wanted to do something about it. I wasn't sure of much, but I did know one thing: I did not want to feel that way any longer. I wasn't upset. I wasn't sad. I was done.

Seven words I said to myself ultimately changed my life. "I will *never* feel this way again."

I didn't care what I had to do or how long it would take. I. Would. Never. Feel. This. Way. Again. These words became the center of my entire being, because these words hold power, assurance, and victory for me. Change sometimes feels so scary, but the day you realize that staying the same is even scarier is the day you will be able to march forward and never look back.

In August of 2014, I elected to have weight-loss surgery. I had convinced myself this was the answer, despite what anyone said to the contrary. I was repeatedly told, "Weight-loss surgery is a tool, and it only works if *you* do."

That statement is so very true, but I was not interested in putting in any work—mentally or physically. I had reached a point where all I knew was that I needed all the external help I could get.

Many people have said, "Weight-loss surgery is the easy way out." Honestly, that's exactly what I was hoping for. I believed it was a foolproof solution that would rid me of my weight problem forever.

After surgery, I faced a harsh reality. Initially I dropped fifty pounds with zero effort, but then I immediately transitioned to my old habits. So that fifty pounds came back on—faster than ever. See, weight-loss surgery can remove part of your stomach, but it cannot fix your habits, your heart, or your broken pieces.

I felt like a weight-loss surgery failure. The surgeon literally removed 80 percent of my stomach, and I still could not manage to stop this cycle that was killing me. I was constantly sick and taking twelve prescription drugs daily just to function. I desperately needed a breakthrough.

I want to pause and take a moment to consider the reasons why so many people struggle to lose weight, even after weight-loss surgery.

Prior to choosing surgery, I often scrolled through social media and looked at weight-loss stories. The first thing I searched for was whether surgery had been involved. If the person had had surgery, I immediately discounted them, thinking they had taken the easy way out.

I desperately needed a breakthrough.

Before long, this "easy way out" felt like the only answer. I wanted my victory so badly, and it seemed impossible not to be successful.

Unfortunately, like so many others, the weight came back, and I was left feeling like a total failure.

During the initial period after weight-loss surgery, you are forced to undergo extreme restrictions. Combined with a period of consuming only liquids, there are severe caloric restrictions. The problem? Your metabolism slows down along with your food intake. Fast-forward a few months, and as old habits creep back in, your metabolism remains slow, which induces weight gain.

Weight-loss surgery doesn't address the heart of the matter.

But most important, weight-loss surgery doesn't address the heart of the matter. There is no way to lose weight long term without attacking your mind-set . . . and no surgery will do that for you.

It's easy to make an assumption that weight-loss surgery always works, because no one is out there posting their failures. The only social media posts you'll see are the successful ones, while those who are still struggling are hiding in the shadows, trying to find the answer they were looking for in the first place.

Thankfully, I eventually discovered the answers I was looking for. These answers are effective, and they last—and my goal is to help you discover the very same answers for yourself and your journey.

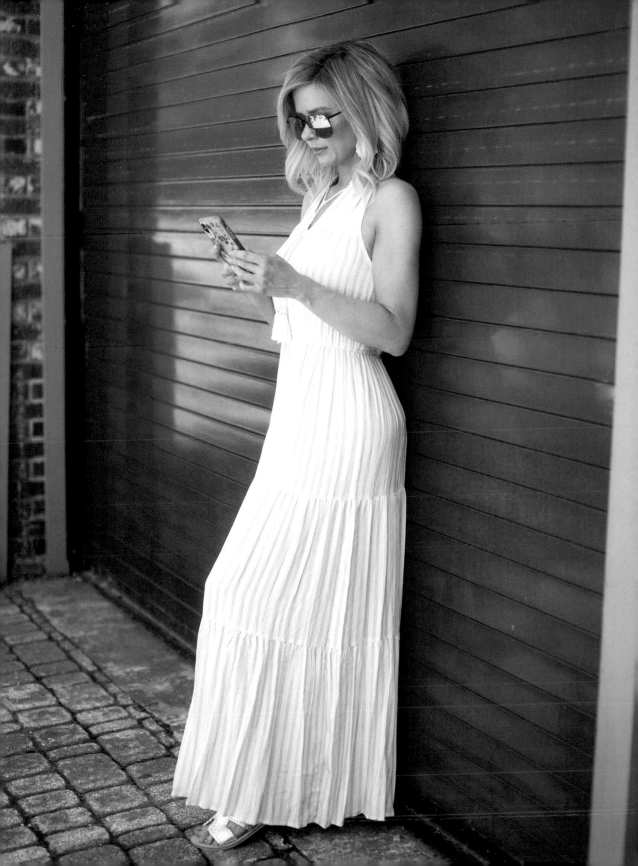

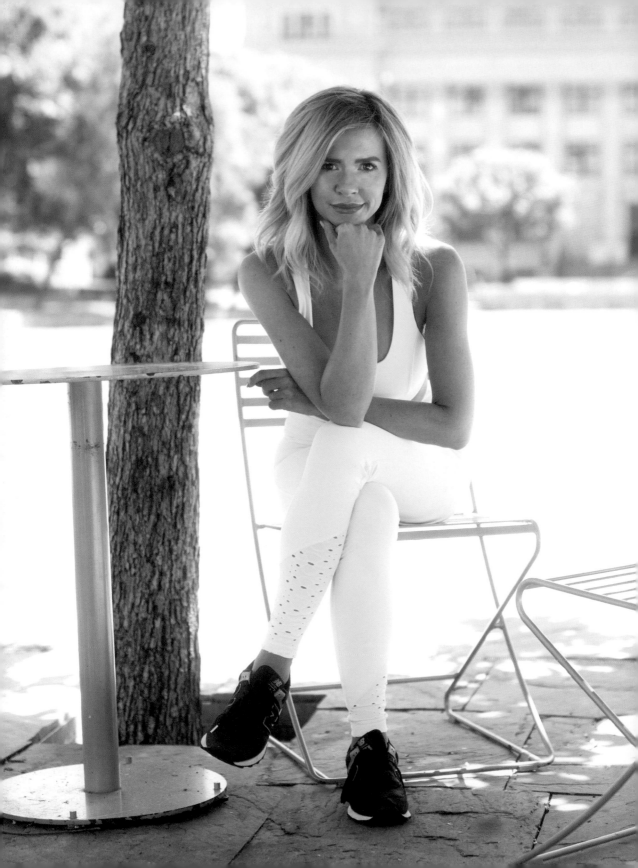

2

THE PATH TO HEALING

It would be so much easier to be hit by an actual truck than to bear the burden of emotional pain. At least when you are hit by a truck, others can see your bruises. You don't have to justify your pain. Your friends and family can be gentle with you as you heal and can see how much you have recovered. If you are having a bad day, it's easy to see why.

But emotional wounds are invisible. They are kept in private under the surface, and if we don't address them, they can spread like an infection that becomes out of control. Others can't see them, and most don't know they are there. Even though others can't see, *you* know the pain you carry, and many of us find unhealthy ways to cope with that pain.

Therefore, I truly believe the only way to achieve successful weight loss is to first attack your mind-set by healing the wounds that can be found at the root of the problem and identifying the foundation of the poor health patterns you've adopted. Your body will *always* follow along

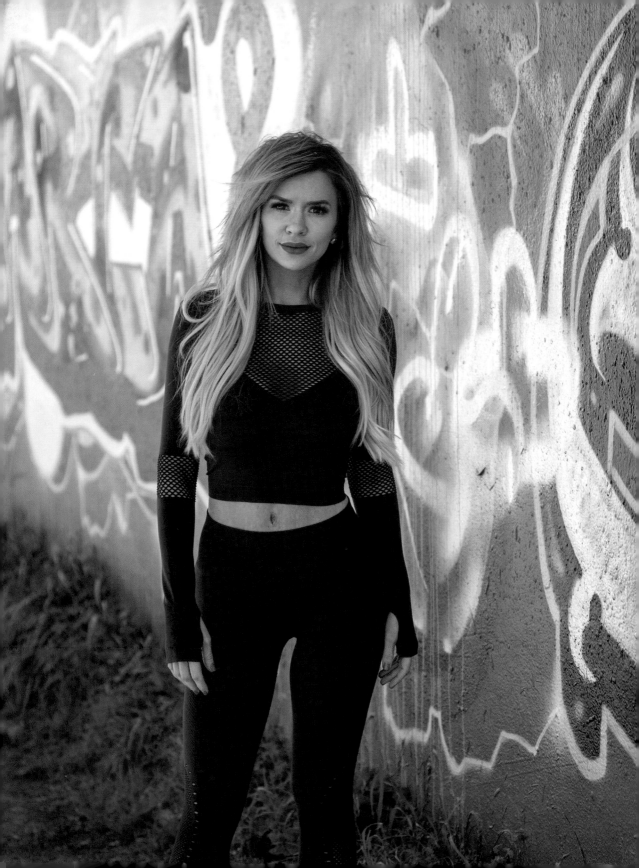

when your mind leads the way. In the following pages, I will describe how I applied each mind-set shift and unlocked the brave spirit that was trapped beneath my weight. The process of transforming how you *think* can feel both challenging and freeing at the same time.

Weight gain stems from many places: heartbreak, parents' divorce (or your own), emotionally and/or physically abusive relationships, loss of a loved one, and the list goes on. Regardless of the emotional trigger, you've stopped putting yourself first, and you probably aren't giving yourself the love and care you deserve. Learning to actively love yourself always comes down to this: true transformation starts in the mind and burns through the body. Take care of your mind first, and a body you love will follow—and stay for good.

> *True transformation starts in the mind and burns through the body.*

As we continue, we will begin to peel back the layers and bad habits that have built up throughout the years as a way to cope with pain from the past. We will expose the warrior hidden beneath and learn to love ourselves again. As we heal from the inside out, we will discover that life was meant to be lived and loved fully.

Why Diets Fail

Each time I began a new diet, I had so much enthusiasm. I would make my plan, throw out all my old food, buy new workout clothes, and take my measurements. I was *sure* this was the time I would succeed. I was convinced nothing could stop me.

However, I was trying to heal myself with the same mind-set that made me sick in the first place. I felt hopeful I could somehow will myself skinny. And while I was never able to will away the pounds, I was eventually able to *think* away the pounds.

The reason diets fail us is because we approach them with the same mind-set we had when we gained the weight. Trust me, I get it. The thought of actually changing your habits for life seems daunting. We think we can beat the system and find an easier way.

*While I was never able to will away the pounds, I was eventually able to **think** away the pounds.*

There are no magical diets, but there are diet styles that work better for some than they do for others. There are also no magical workouts. But there is a way—between adjusting your mind-set and creating a plan to work with *your* lifestyle—to find the transformation you are looking for. Statistics tell us that 65 percent of women who lose weight will gain that weight back in less than three years. It is my purpose in life to lower that percentage, and it starts with *you*.

In the chapters to come, I will explain the transition of mind-sets that needs to happen before you can begin to change your actions. As you come to understand this process, you will uncover pieces of yourself you didn't even know existed and a strength to overcome you haven't found previously. Then I will walk you through the diet I followed (and still follow to this day) as well as show you simple workouts that will maximize your results and serve as a consistent fitness foundation on this journey.

Some days you will want to throw in the towel, but stay with me. Diamonds are made under pressure, so don't resist when the hard days come. Stay the course.

The All-or-Nothing Mentality

I am an extremist by nature. Maybe you can relate. This character trait—or flaw, depending on who you're asking—is woven deep into my being. When channeled the right way, I can use this trait to move mountains. But when channeled the wrong way, I find myself in a debilitating cycle of self-doubt, self-loathing, and self-deprecation.

The all-or-nothing mentality is well-known to extremists, but most of us are familiar with it on some level. We feel if we are not all in, we have to be all out. Rarely do we feel comfortable in the middle.

This is the first mind-set shift that must change.

For a good example of this mind-set shift, let's take a look at how our motivation tends to play out when it comes to weight loss. *Motivation* is what you feel when you first start a diet. You are full of excitement and energy and want to be *all in*. You plan your meals and your workouts, and you are convinced this is the time it's going to work for you. This is the time you are finally going to do what you say you are going to do: lose weight!

> *Diamonds are made under pressure, so don't resist when the hard days come.*

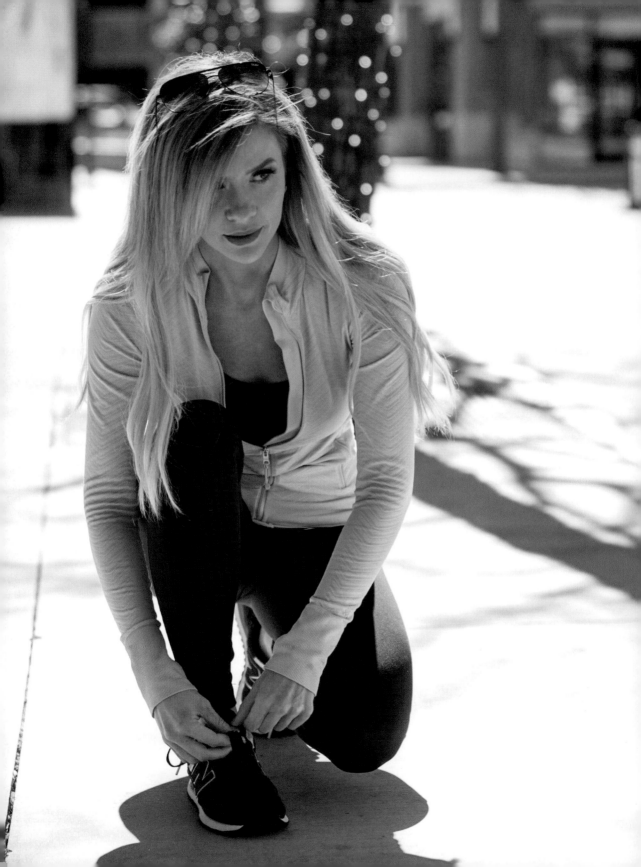

Then life happens. Stress begins piling up and temptation seems to come at you from every direction. The motivation and willpower you once felt is lost, and you cave in and eat something—or many things—that are not part of your meal plan.

At this point you think to yourself: *Well, despite all my preparation and initial motivation, I screwed up. I guess I'll try to start over again tomorrow. Or Monday. Or New Year's.* This vicious cycle repeats itself time and time again, and you always end up back where you started.

To change this mind-set, you simply need to change what you tell yourself in the moments when you acknowledge you've screwed up. When you cheat on your diet plan, you must say the following to yourself: *That's okay. I forgive myself. I'm going to get back on track this minute!*

At first this will be a struggle to embrace—and that's okay! Please don't be so hard on yourself. The first time you decide to rebound, you might not get back on your plan fully for three days. No problem! But the next time you step off the path toward better health, make it your goal to get back on in two days . . . then one day. If you keep closing the gap, you will discover that it becomes easier to step right back on your path when you find yourself off course.

> *To change this mind-set, you simply need to change what you tell yourself in the moments when you acknowledge you've screwed up.*

Chains of Habit

There is a quote attributed to Samuel Johnson: "The chains of habit are too weak to be felt until they are too strong to be broken." When applied to a weight-loss journey, this quote can go one of two ways.

Our habits are the foundation of everything we do, and our success literally relies on them. When we do not see the victories in our life that we wish to see, there's a strong possibility this means our bad habits are outweighing the good. My goal is to help you change what you *do* on a regular, habitual basis so that you can uncover who you are meant to become.

During my downward spiral, I never noticed the bad habits that had crept into my life until they consumed me. Some of those habits included:

- Resorting to food when feeling stressed or depressed
- Resorting to medication to control my emotions
- Not taking care of myself
- Not eating right
- Not exercising

I could go on for *days* giving you an unending list of unhealthy habits that were collectively breaking me. These habits had slowly become ingrained throughout all areas of my life, and I had become their slave. I was not the master of my decisions but a victim to my habits.

That same Samuel Johnson quote can also be applied to the other side of the spectrum. As you begin to replace old, unhealthy habits with new,

I WOULD
GRAB TWO
DONUTS
WITHOUT
EVEN
THINKING.

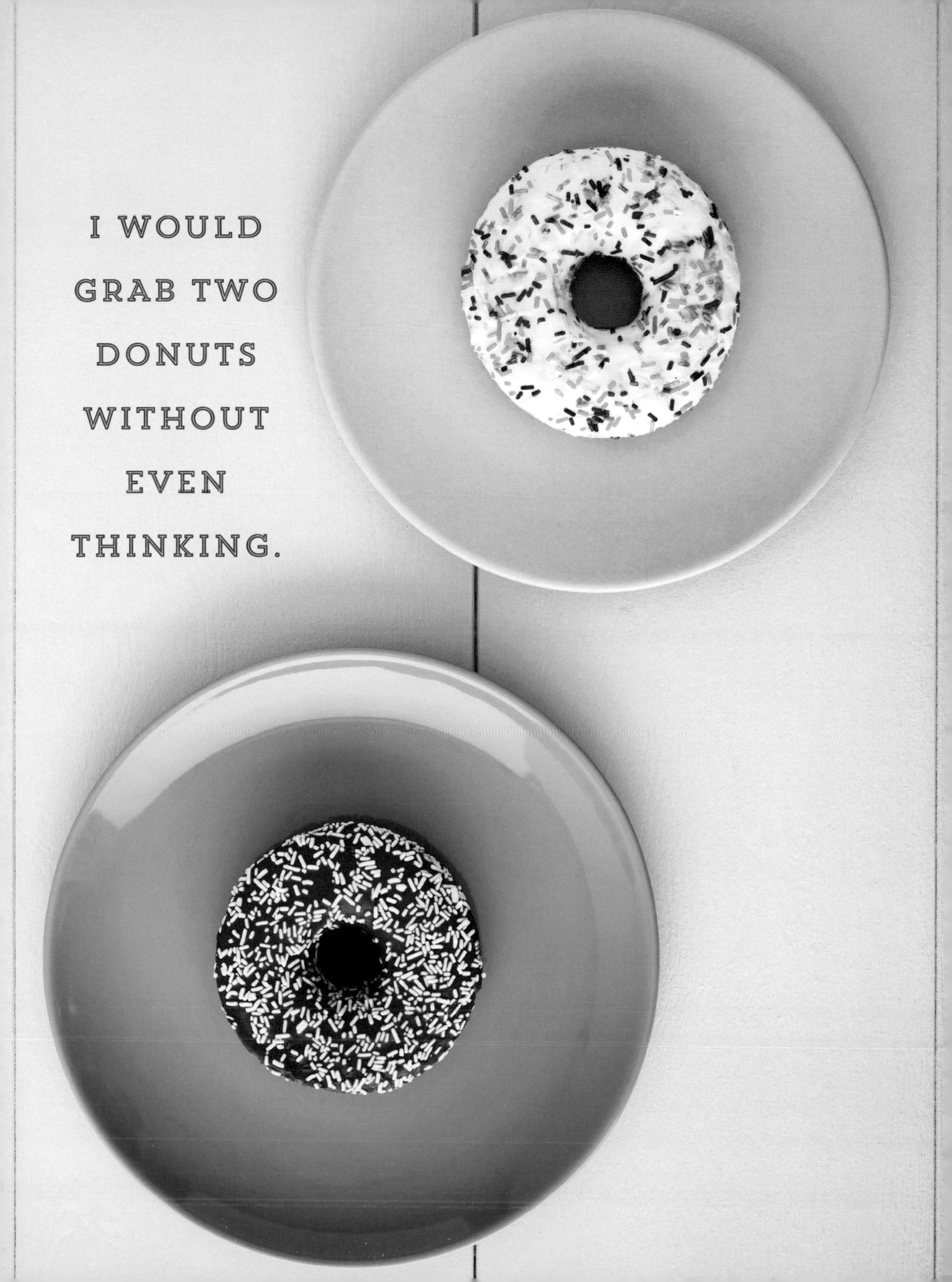

healthy ones, you will not even notice when the new habits have become routine. One day you will simply realize that doing something healthy has become a conscious choice you're making.

I was not the master of my decisions but a victim to my habits.

Before, I never could resist donuts in the office. When I walked into my breakroom at work, I would grab two donuts without even thinking. Now that I have replaced my old habits, the temptation of a donut sounds more like this in my mind: *Wow, those donuts look tasty. Should I have one? Actually, last time I had a donut it didn't really satisfy me, and I felt terrible all day. I had no energy and felt nauseated. Hmm. I think I'll pass this time. I'm up to too many things today.*

These days, my new habits win out because I have practiced them for years and have improved my ability to stick to them. I'll share how I began shifting my own mind-set with a two-part exercise.

Habits are everything, and the Mindshift Exercise on the following page is powerful, allowing you to become present to both your conscious and unconscious habits—especially the ones that sabotage your progress. It's important to pay attention to the ones we automatically default to when we're too tired to think. However, by consciously choosing a new habit to put in its place, and practicing every day, this new healthy habit eventually becomes an automatic part of our routine. Cultivating habits and routines doesn't mean that we go through life mindlessly, however. In fact, this exercise is about intentionally and mindfully cultivating new habits that set us up for success.

MINDSHIFT EXERCISE

STEP 1: WRITE DOWN YOUR CURRENT HABITS

To change your habits, first identify the habits and thought patterns that keep you in chains. Write down a list of your current unhealthy habits to get a good picture of why you are where you are. This could include:

- Skipping meals until you're starving and unable to make healthy choices
- Caving in to office treats
- Stopping by the drive-thru on the way home before dinner
- Eating sweets as a reward for working out
- Having an extra glass of wine for getting through a hard day

STEP 2: WRITE DOWN YOUR NEW HABITS

The next step is to write down your plan to replace those habits with better ones. Some of my new habits include:

- Daily time with God
- Daily exercise for at least ten minutes
- Planning my meals the night prior
- Daily affirmations
- Drinking a glass of water as soon as I wake up

This is not a one-time exercise. This must be a living, breathing list that evolves. As you become who you were meant to be, cross off old habits and replace them with new ones.

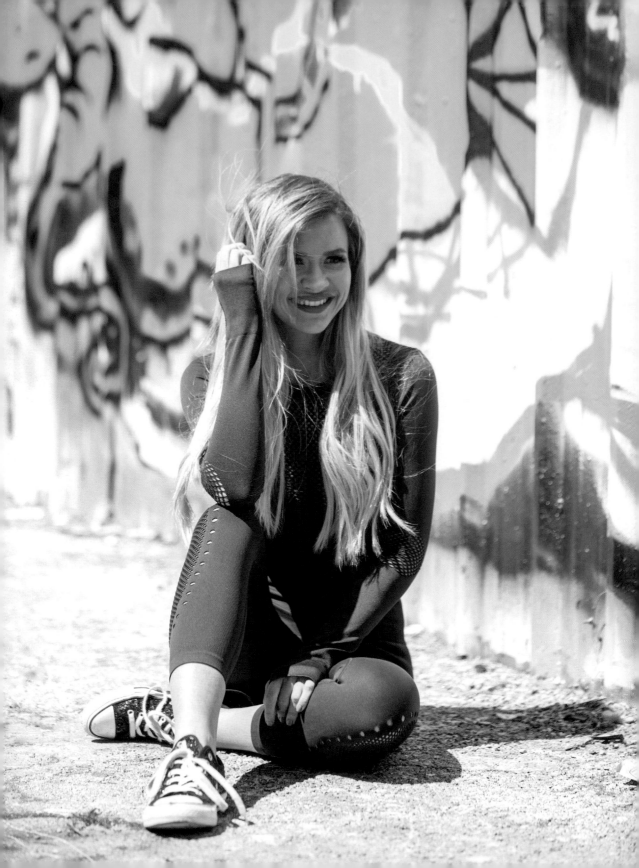

YOU ARE NOT A NUMBER

The scale is a liar.

I want you to say it out loud: "The scale . . . is a *liar.*"

We are living in a time when it is particularly easy to define ourselves by the numbers and measurements society says we should have. Some of those numbers include:

- The number on the scale

- Our credit score

- The amount of money we have in the bank

- How much our car costs

- How much our home costs

- How many likes we get on a social media post

We feel valuable only when our numbers meet societal expectations. But you are worth far more than any number, especially the one on the scale.

Here are the things the scale cannot measure:

- How caring you are
- What a good spouse, parent, sibling, aunt or uncle, friend, or daughter or son you are
- How good you are at your job
- How in tune your heart is to serving others
- How beautiful you are inside and out
- The difference you make in someone's life

The scale is *nothing* more than the gravitational relationship between you and the ground. I have a feeling if the number on the scale remained the *same*, but you woke up with your dream life and goal body, you wouldn't give one hoot what number showed up.

The real question is: What else should you be measuring?

Now, it is true that the scale is a literal measure of weight. But the real question is: What *else* should you be measuring?

When I first started my weight-loss journey, I borrowed a two-piece bikini from a friend and took the most mortifying photos I have ever laid eyes on. I could see the misery in my own face as I took the pictures. I was *so* embarrassed of these pictures that I purchased a password-protected vault app, on my phone, to ensure that *no one* would *ever* see them. (It's funny, because millions of people have now seen these pictures as part of the before-and-after shot for my business.)

THE
SCALE
IS A
LIAR.

Taking "before" photos is particularly difficult because it requires you to be brutally honest with yourself. You know you aren't where you want to be and taking an unflattering photo to remind you of that place can be downright heartbreaking. But I promise you will not regret doing this. One day you will look back and cherish these photos as a reminder of how far you have come and of the mountains God has helped you move.

Taking photos along your journey is a powerful way to stay on track. There were so many times the scale just wasn't moving, but as I took updated pictures, I saw massive changes. This is one of the reasons why the scale doesn't matter when it comes to measuring your progress.

Another great indicator of progress is using a simple tape measure to take various body measurements. You can write each of these down in a fitness journal, or you can download one of the many phone apps that allow you to record and track your body measurements. Typically, the best places to measure are bust, chest, waist, hips, thighs, calves, upper arm, and forearm. You will find, many times, that the scale has moved only a few pounds. But by maintaining a progress chart and measuring once a week or once a month, you'll see you're losing inches and your measurements have changed significantly.

It does not define you.

All in all, my advice to you is this: do not allow yourself to become a slave to the scale. Do not allow the scale to dictate how your day will go. And most of all, do not let that lying scale add or take away value from who you are. It's just a number. It does not define you.

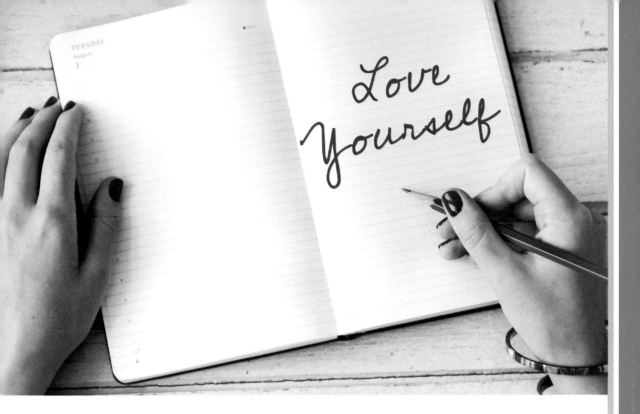

Learn to Love Yourself Again

Four years ago I wanted to go to a restaurant for dinner. I'd had a very stressful day at my job in corporate America and was at the end of my proverbial rope. The only thought flooding my mind was, *brisket enchiladas will solve everything*. And at that time, I believed that to be true.

I pulled up to the restaurant, and there was a forty-five-minute wait. This was not a problem for me, because there was no way I was going to walk away from the food I had prescribed myself to heal me of my stress. When my turn finally came, the hostess called my name, and I proceeded to the booth. This restaurant was set up with all of the tables in the middle and all of the booths surrounded those tables forming a large circle. Every restaurant patron could see each other.

As I approached my table, I eyeballed which side of the booth was bigger. I always picked the bigger side because one of my deepest fears was not fitting in the booth. This was the day one of my deepest fears would become reality.

> ## Then came the worst part: I got stuck.

My eyeballing wasn't too helpful, as the booth situation was pretty grim. Turns out, both sides of the booth were quite narrow. And to be fair, even at my current healthy weight, it would have been tight. Alas, I tried to squeeze in anyway. Then came the worst part: I got stuck. I literally tried to force myself in so hard that I became wedged between the seat and the table. The host had to grab my arms and help pull me out of the predicament I had found myself in.

I. Was. Mortified.

Now I was faced with two choices, and both were humiliating:

1. Go back to the front and wait for a table I could fit in.
2. Tuck my head down in shame and leave.

As I walked back to the entryway, I heard the host say to a coworker, "She was too fat to fit in the booth, so we need to give her the next available table."

I was too fat to fit in the booth. Nine words that haunt me—to this day—every time I approach a booth at a restaurant.

Now, you're probably thinking, *You left immediately, right?!* But I couldn't. I came for stress-reducing enchiladas, and my stress level had now doubled. I wasn't leaving without filling the emptiness inside. I needed those enchiladas.

I was stuck in a cycle in which I did not love myself enough to trust I could overcome my stress without relying on my most powerful crutch: food. I couldn't see it at the time, but all the negative mind-set habits I was repeating internally were breaking me down further and further. I no longer felt worth it. I was ashamed of who I had become. I didn't even recognize myself anymore.

In order to fix what is going on in our lives, we *must* fix what is going on in our hearts—and that begins with first fully understanding and embracing self-love. You were created in the image of God, who deeply loves and values you. The more you embrace this truth and learn ways to prioritize your health as a result, the more you have to give to others in your life, and the more energy you have to dedicate to your family, work, or any other life purpose or pursuit. When you fill yourself up first, you no longer pour from an empty cup. For me, having a strong faith in God keeps my cup full.

IN ORDER TO FIX
WHAT IS GOING ON
IN OUR LIVES, WE
MUST FIX WHAT
IS GOING ON IN
OUR HEARTS.

You might not know exactly where this cycle began. You might be asking yourself, "*Why did I stop loving myself in the first place?*" For a lot of us, the un-loving process begins with putting others first and failing to examine or tend to our own needs. When we focus too much on the instinct to act as caretakers, slowly but surely we neglect to do the things we need to do in order to ensure *we* are taken care of. The key phrase here is *too much*.

I had reached a place where I put my job, loved ones, friends, and my brother with special needs before myself. Every time I put their needs above mine, I lost a tiny piece of myself. Over and over I did this, repeatedly telling myself my needs could wait and never taking the time to make sure I had what I needed.

Most of us feel selfish if we even entertain the idea of putting ourselves first, especially when someone needs us. And even when they don't necessarily require special time or attention, we have trained our minds that self-care is some form of narcissism and should be avoided.

But here is my question to you: If you neglect yourself, are you really giving 100 percent to anyone at all?

It's easy to *feel* as though we are giving our entire effort to the things we care about, but the reality is we are pouring from an empty cup. We can't give our best because we don't have our best to give.

Self-love is a choice.

Self-love is a choice. Prioritizing your health is a decision you must make daily in order to fulfill your life's calling and be able to pour into others' lives as well. So take a moment every morning to tell yourself you *are* worth it and to remind yourself of what you are doing this for—to become the best version of who God created you to be.

I want to walk you through an exercise I implemented into my daily routine that has helped me truly reconnect with myself and come to a place of self-love. It's funny, because we are often quick to come down on ourselves for all of the things we are not, and we fail to see all of the wonderful things we are.

Just like God does, our bodies are going to keep supporting us even on the days we don't deserve it.

Our mind tells us things like:

- You aren't pretty enough.
- Your thighs are too thick.
- You look bad in everything.
- You aren't in good enough shape.

But here's the reality: your body is beautiful and incredible and still fights for you every single day, even when you haven't always shown it the love it deserves. Our bodies are created in God's image. Just like God does, our bodies are going to keep supporting us even on the days we don't deserve it.

Here's the truth about your body:

- You have a heart that still beats for you.
- You have lungs that still breathe for you.
- You have legs that still carry you where you want to go.
- You have arms that allow you to pet your animals or pick up your children.

SELF-LOVE EXERCISE

1. Pull yourself into a quiet space where you are free from distraction. Take a deep breath in and imagine you are inhaling peace and happiness; then exhale and imagine you are letting go of doubt, guilt, and shame.

2. With your eyes closed, place your hand over your heart. Feel it beating for you. This is a great opportunity to remember that even when you don't take care of your body, your heart still beats. It isn't giving up on you. Out loud, say, "Thank you for beating for me every moment of every day."

3. Keeping your eyes closed and your hand in place, feel your lungs as they take in air for you. Take another deep breath. Those lungs still believe in you! They support you every single day and bring oxygen into your body. Your lungs want you to thrive. Out loud, say, "Thank you for breathing for me. Thank you for not giving up on me."

I encourage you to practice this exercise with all different body parts. For my mamas out there, place your hands on your belly and thank your tummy for carrying your children for you. You will likely be so surprised at how life-altering it can be when we transition our thoughts from rejecting our body to being thankful for it.

There are so many precious things about our bodies, and we have to learn to practice being thankful for them. After years of entertaining deprecating thoughts, it will probably feel unnatural to start appreciating your body for what it is. However, I want to encourage you to find five minutes each day to practice the Self-Love Exercise.

Another great step you can take to start this process is by doing daily affirmations. I'll be honest—at first, the thought of reading something motivational and dwelling on it all day seemed really silly to me. Even though it felt awkward, I decided to give it a try. What did I have to lose? Every morning I pick a phrase, quote, or Bible verse that motivates me, and I write it down on a piece of paper. Multiple times throughout the day, I pick up that piece of paper and read it out loud.

Our lives are a direct reflection of what we say and think about ourselves.

What I've found is that our lives are a direct reflection of what we say and think about ourselves. When you start to speak positivity over yourself, you train your brain into believing your words are true. Do this for long enough, and you will actually *believe* that what you are saying is true.

After my assault, my self-worth was at an all-time low, and this led to the perpetual cycle of un-loving myself. I never believed I could come to a place where I understood my value or my worth. The mountain in front of me felt *much* bigger than the God inside of me, and I thought I would never break free from the prison of my mind that held me captive. I want to give you this encouragement: after all of those years of struggle, I was able to do it, and you can too! Together, we will start walking through mind-set shifts that can help you find the hero within and start showing them the love they've been needing for so long.

MOST > NOW

The new habits you are working to create and build on, as you read this book, are habits that will help you for the rest of your life. Weight loss is not a one-and-done practice. If you change your habits for only a short time, you will always see short-term results.

Daily affirmations have become an important part of my practice and success. I encourage you to find one that resonates with you, write it down, post it where you can see it, and recite it every day. Some of my favorite daily affirmations include:

"I am fearfully and wonderfully made" (Psalm 139:14).

"I am worthy of giving and receiving love."

"I can either give *up*, give *in*, or give it *my all*."

Recently, I found myself in a predicament. Over the Thanksgiving holiday, I allowed myself to splurge and eat outside of my normal diet. The tasty treats I devoured made me feel *amazing* for exactly six minutes. But then my body felt like it had been hit by a Mack truck. I had a tummy ache, a headache, and I wanted to retreat to my bed.

In the days that followed, my old habits tried to come back into play. I found myself following my nutrition guidelines all day and then blowing it in the evening. After years of feeling so strong in my habits, one day of delectable delights had me frazzled.

It was time to get back to the basics and think myself through this. Every time I craved something sugary and sweet, I asked myself one question: *Is this contributing to what I want* most *or to what I want* now?

Is this contributing to what I want most or to what I want now?

What I want most is to look and feel incredible—and to be able to love others well as a result of prioritizing my own emotional and physical health. I want to operate at my highest potential without allowing food to have control over me. I certainly do *not* want to go back to the old version of myself.

You may not know yet what you want most, and that's okay. But I want to walk you through a few exercises that will allow you to dedicate some focused time to help you determine who you want to become and discover what you envision for your life.

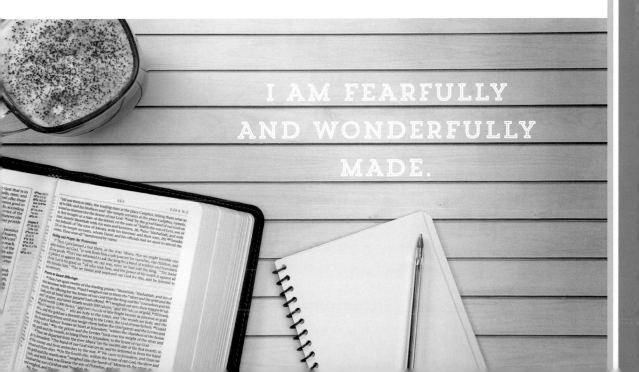

I AM FEARFULLY AND WONDERFULLY MADE.

DEFINE YOUR WHY

It's time to grab your notebook again for the next part of our journey.

STEP 1: WRITE OUT YOUR "WHY"

When it comes to a weight-loss journey, the most important question you can ask yourself is: "Why am I really doing this?"

Your initial response may be: *"Because I want to be skinny!"*

However, I want to challenge you. If the only "why" motivating your journey is aesthetic, you need to look deeper beneath the surface and find a reason that will sustain you. Most of us *think* we want to look a certain way, but the reality is that most of us want to *feel* a certain way.

I was sick and tired of being sick and tired. I was fed up with my depression and all the thoughts in my head that made my giants seem bigger than me. I wanted to walk into a room and not ask myself whether I was the biggest person there.

I wanted to be happy. I wanted my life back. I wanted to find me.

Diving in and understanding what you are truly seeking is the first step to finding out what you are chasing after. Additionally, this process is ever-evolving. Your "why" today may be very different from your "why" a year from now. So take the time to do this exercise every few months, and start by looking back at what you've written down in the past. You might be surprised to see how much your mind-set has shifted from the beginning of your journey.

STEP 2: WRITE OUT WHO YOU WANT TO BE

This exercise feels a lot like the timeless question: "What do you want to be when you grow up?"

But this step in the process turned out to be a game changer without me even recognizing it initially.

I want you to stand in front of a mirror and look into your own eyes. Then ask yourself the following questions:

1. Who is [your name here]?
2. What defines him/her?
3. What kind of person is he/she?
4. What kind of person is he/she married to?
5. What kind of job does he/she have?
6. What kind of house does he/she live in?
7. What does he/she do to make a difference in the lives of other people?

I first did this exercise in the spring of 2016. I was recently divorced and I felt lost. I was halfway through my weight-loss journey, but still lacked direction. I didn't know who I was at this point in my life.

When I first wrote out this exercise, I said the following to myself in the mirror:

Christine Carter is a loving woman who wants to show other people how to change their lives. She does this by consistently leading by example, supporting them, and offering advice. She is single, for now, but eventually finds a partner who will chase after God and after life with her. She lives in a cool high-rise in downtown Dallas, drives a white BMW, and is a director at her company.

The funny thing is, I totally forgot about this exercise and went on with my life. Eight months later I found this piece of paper in a drawer . . . as I was packing to move to my high-rise . . . in my white BMW. I was dumbfounded. I had no idea the *power* that writing out a vision could hold, even when it wasn't something I was focusing on. Just the act of writing out your dreams and visions has incredible power.

Fast-forward to today and I still do this exercise every three to four months. As you continue to grow and evolve, it is critical that you continue to repeat these steps so you never become stagnant in your personal growth.

STEP 3: DRAW OUT YOUR MAP

So often we want to change but have no real strategy or plan of attack to make it happen. We will dive into the diet and workout portion of your map in a later chapter, but first and foremost, for true and lasting change, you need a mind-set map. The map is a pathway to success that you can refer to daily, something you can always turn to when you're confronted or struggling. You can have either a "fixed mind-set" or a "growth mind-set." The exercises in this book help you create the latter.

When writing out your map, you want to refer back to the unhealthy habits you'd like to kick to the curb. Then make a plan, for every day, to start filling yourself up with healthy habits instead.

Here are a few of the healthy habits I began implementing:

1. Daily affirmations
2. Daily reading of my "why"
3. Daily reading of a personal development book chapter
4. Swapping my pop music for worship/motivational music

It is critical that you revisit these steps often. Do not allow this to be a one-time exercise you never think about again. In the beginning, I recommend reminding yourself daily *why* you want to change, *who* you want to become, and *what* steps you are taking to make sure you succeed.

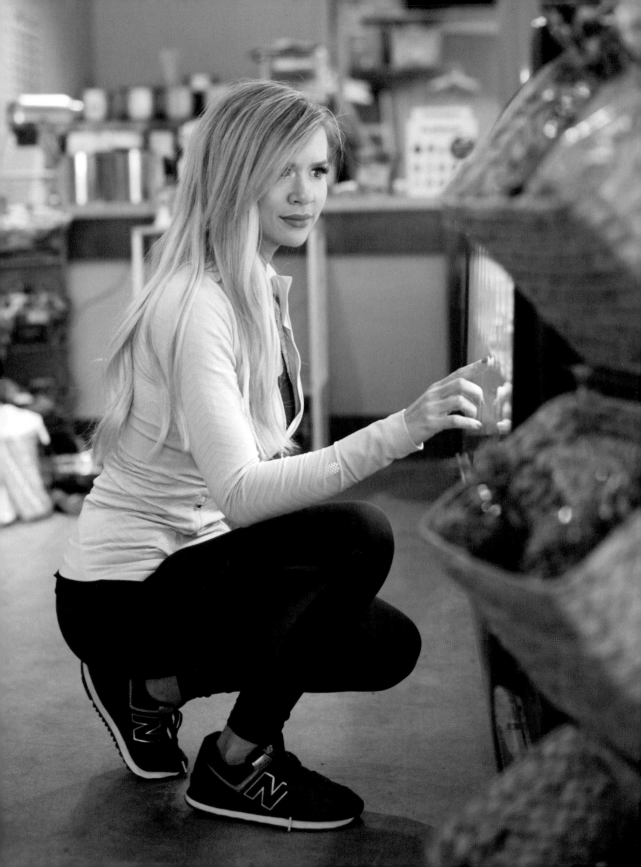

4

BUILDING BLOCKS

We have already discussed the all-or-nothing mentality that can keep us in a cycle of highs and lows, but I want to break this down a bit further. Often when we begin a new weight-loss plan, we believe we must get *everything* right from the word *go* in order to succeed.

Have you ever heard the famous question: "How do you eat an elephant?" The answer: one bite at a time. If you truly are committed to making changes that will last, you have to break this down into smaller bite-size pieces.

This concept was so challenging for me to understand. I constantly felt frustrated that I could not just . . . change. I wanted so badly to be in a different place in my journey that I would try to make all the changes at once.

What I later learned is that it is better to master small changes, one by one, rather than continuing to fail at some perceived level of perfection we try so hard to achieve all at once. Progress is better than perfection—any

I STARTED WITH BREAKFAST.

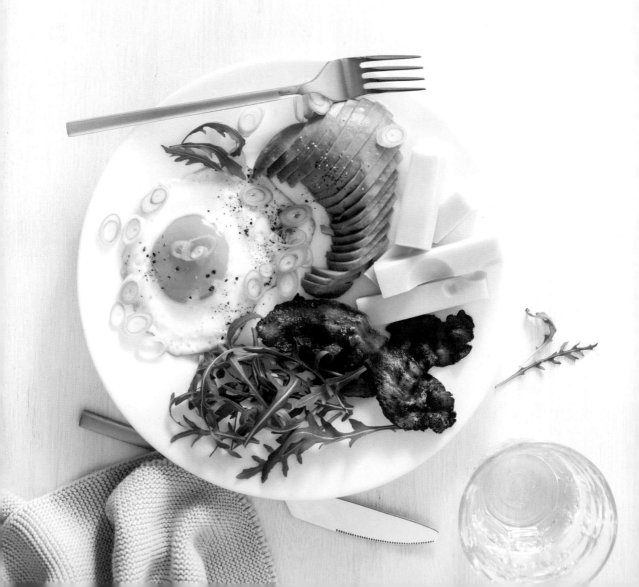

day of the week. During my journey I found a quote attributed to psychologist Émile Coué that I repeated to myself over and over: "Every day, in every way, I'm getting better and better." This does not mean that every day I will be *perfect*. Some days I might not even be *great*. But each day, in each way, I am taking steps toward improvement.

I started with breakfast. I decided I could do anything else I wanted with the rest of my day as long as I ate the right thing for breakfast. This is a very helpful trick for those suffering from a binge eating disorder and for anyone whose struggle with weight is defined by a lack of discipline or self-control. It tricks your mind by telling it, *"Later . . . just not right now."* After mastering the ability to slay my breakfast, I added another building block—my morning snack.

From there, I kept adding more building blocks until all of these things became my entire daily routine.

Long-Term Habits and Short-Term Goals

Having goals is good, and creating habits is *great*, but what if there is more to the story? So often we set massive, incredible goals when we first start out, but do not focus on the short-term habits to get us there. You may say, "I want to lose fifty pounds, and I am going to follow XYZ diet until I get there." But when we do this, we end up focusing more on the long-term goal when it is the short-term habits where we lose the battle, preventing us from winning the war.

After losing one hundred pounds, I was more fed up than ever. I struggled with the "Are we there yet?" syndrome. I felt stuck in the gap between where I had been and where I wanted to be. I would look at pictures of myself and desperately try to see the differences. I became a slave to the scale. I worked so hard and still hated the skin I was in. I was losing motivation . . . and fast.

During this process, I had to change my outlook. By building only short-term goals and focusing only on the big picture, I found myself frustrated. When temptation struck, my big goals felt impossible and my short-term habits were not yet built to last.

> I became a slave to the scale.

I got past this mental plateau by adjusting my mind-set on the amount of weight I wanted to lose. I no longer had a goal weight in mind but instead focused on a goal *life*. I created a short-term goal to lose just five pounds and was determined to become really good at losing five pounds over and over. By setting these small goals, my motivation grew and grew like a snowball rolling down a hill, and my mind-set became more positive than ever.

Just like habits, our personal mind-set is a critical component to our success—not just with weight loss, but with any important goal we set for ourselves. Take time to go deep with the Mind-Setting Exercise on the following pages, and revisit this anytime you're struggling or feeling stuck.

MIND-SETTING EXERCISE

This is a great place to get into action. Just thinking through your goals isn't enough to help you reach them.

STEP 1: WRITE YOUR SHORT-TERM GOALS

Pull out your pen and notebook and jot down your short-term goals. Remember, this is an evolving exercise that should be revisited often.

Here are a few of mine when I first started:

- Lose five pounds.
- Drop one pant size.
- Bc able to walk up one flight of stairs without feeling winded.

I also had to change my view of short-term habits, because short-term habits will never last. I was in this for the long haul. We know that the sum of our life comes down to our daily habits. If I do XYZ for one month and see great success, I will not be able to maintain that success if I discontinue the habits. I didn't need habits for weight loss. I needed habits for *life*.

STEP 2: WRITE YOUR NEW HEALTHY HABITS

Write down what habits you could put into practice, beginning today. These are some of the initial habits I put into practice:

- Eat a healthy breakfast every day.
- Walk for twenty minutes a day, five days a week, on my lunch break.
- Read one chapter each day of a personal development book. (*You're Going to Be Okay* by Holley Gerth is a great book to start with.)

When you find yourself in the mind trap of "Are we there yet?" I want you to shift your focus to how far you have come and revisit your lists of short-term goals and habits. You might find that while you haven't reached your final destination, you've become really good at meeting small goals along the way and forming short-term habits that will eventually become permanent habits. Or you might find you need to reevaluate these lists and make changes that will set you up for more success. When your positive results don't seem to be coming as quickly or as easily as you think they should, remember that there is beauty in the process. Strength is found in truly learning about and understanding yourself.

Trust the Process

In the pages to come, we will take what we have learned about shifting our mind-sets and begin examining the diet and workout portion of the plan. But before we go there, I want to spend a moment with you to talk about learning to *trust the process*.

When I first started this plan, I wanted immediate results. *I've been on a diet for thirty minutes. Why am I not skinny yet?* I look back on this and laugh, because I was not mentally in a place to be able to maintain my dream body just yet.

The harsh reality is that for most of us, if we woke up with our dream body and dream life today, we would not have the discipline and habits in place to maintain them. It's just like the lottery effect. According to the National Endowment for Financial Education, 70 percent of people who win the lottery or receive a large financial windfall will go completely broke within a few years. The same mind-set applies to weight loss. Just as most lottery winners do not have the understanding and discipline to maintain their newfound surplus of wealth, you do not have what it takes to stay healthy if your building blocks and long-term habits are not yet in place.

Trusting the process is more about trusting in your own ability to stick to it no matter what. When I started this process, the scale did not move *one ounce* for twenty-one days. *Twenty-one days!* I would ugly-cry

> I was not mentally in a place to be able to maintain my dream body just yet.

I've been on a diet for thirty minutes. Why am I not skinny yet?

my eyes out on my way to work every morning because I wasn't trusting the process. I wanted instant results for a journey that was going to take much longer than a single month.

Nevertheless, I pressed on. And I went on to lose over 150 pounds on the exact plan I will share with you in the chapters that follow. When I combined the right foods, the right workouts, and the *daily* focus on improving my mind and heart, I found the exact results I was looking for. Most important, I found myself. The self that was there all along. I just needed to dig her out of the hole she had buried herself in.

As you begin your journey, you will undoubtedly have moments when you don't feel like the process is working. In those frustrating moments, I pray that the quiet whisper of "trust the process" remains in your ear. As you build your ability to stay consistent, follow your map, and get back on track when you have a misstep, you will uncover the warrior within, lose the weight that has tied you down for years, and find the authentic *you* that you are meant to be.

In the next part of the book, we'll look at various aspects of the keto-genic diet. Whether you're well-versed or brand-new new to this diet, we'll discuss how to make this healthy lifestyle work for you.

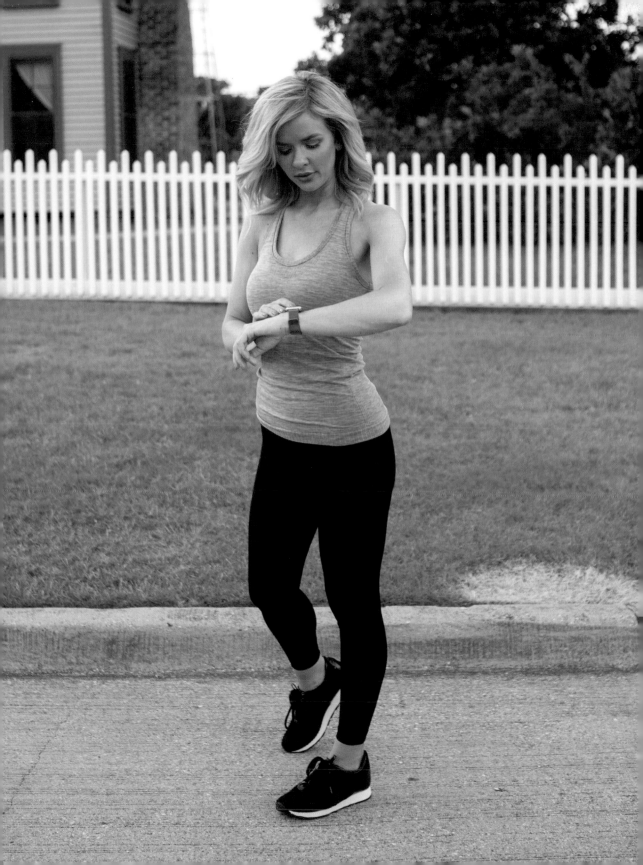

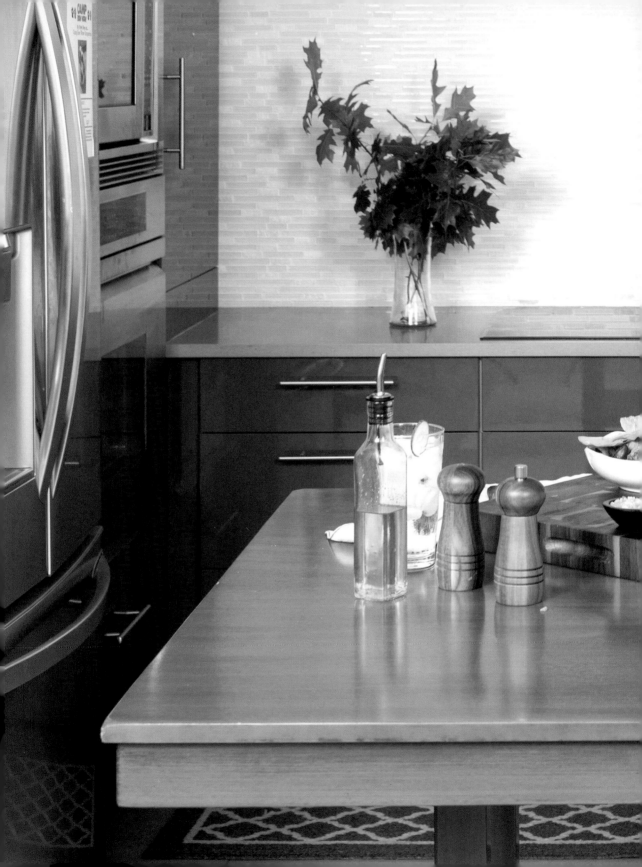

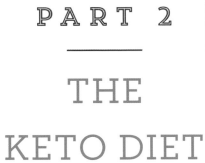

PART 2

THE KETO DIET

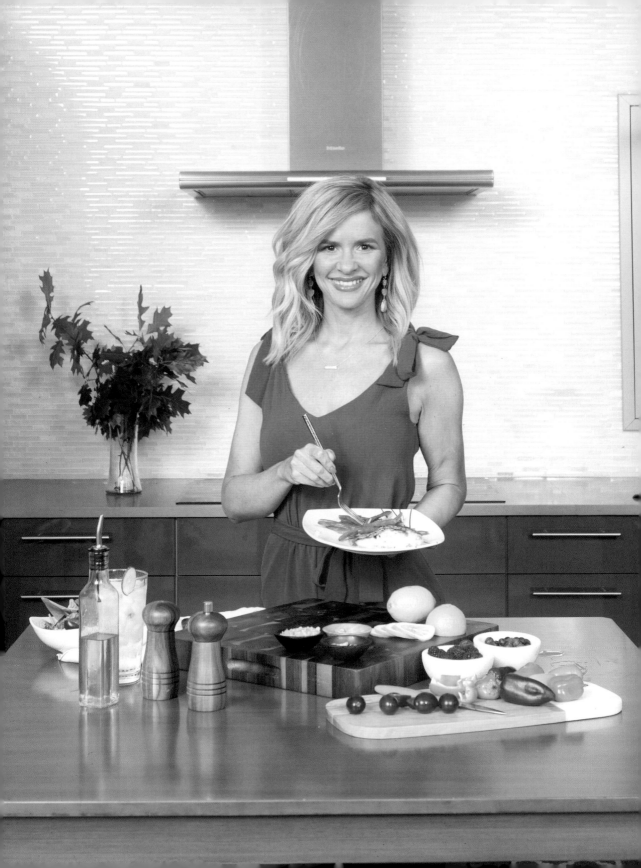

5

APPROACHING A
KETO LIFESTYLE

Chances are that if you have done any research on diets, the ketogenic (keto) diet has popped up more than once. With it, you might find lots of confusion around the topics of: What is keto, exactly? Is it good for me? Can I do it long term?

What makes this diet style confusing is that you could ask ten keto experts to define the ketogenic diet and get ten different answers—and they would all be right. That's because science is not static. We learn new things each day. As I dive into the ketogenic diet, I am offering you my personal approach to this lifestyle. This is the approach that worked for me personally, and it's the one I have used to work with thousands of clients around the world.

Have you ever seen the girl at the gym who *kills* it consistently every

> *I wanted to lose the weight so badly, but I didn't know where to begin.*

day but doesn't drop any weight? That girl was me. Put me on a treadmill, and I would walk for an hour at a moderate pace. Come back a year later, and I'm ten pounds heavier and still walking away.

When I began my weight-loss journey, I was hopeful that perhaps I could eat whatever I wanted and work it off at the gym. I hate to be the bearer of bad news, but you can't outrun your fork. I was a fast-food fanatic. I didn't like to cook, and the only meals I was willing to whip up had enough calories to feed an entire army. My health habits were a wreck. I wanted to lose the weight *so badly*, but I didn't know where to begin.

Diets always felt so scary and daunting to me. I would see girls with a "goal body" eating greens and salmon, and I never could picture myself actually enjoying those things. I always wondered if they pretended to like those foods or if they were insane. I didn't really care either way; I just wanted to look like them.

When I first started, nutrition was the last thing on my mind. If someone started talking to me about nutrients, my mind would begin daydreaming about apple fritters. I didn't want to be *healthy* . . . I wanted to be *thin*.

Through this process, I realized that most of us aren't going to go from a "Frappuccino and french fry fiend" to a "kale salad killer" overnight. (For the record, I still hate kale.) I had to let go of the notion that I had to get it all perfect and, instead, focus on *progression*.

Through the phases in this section, I will walk you through my own personal journey of what I call transitional wellness. From a diet perspective, we will first attack any underlying sugar addiction and begin focusing on the following main food categories (or macronutrients): fats, proteins, and carbs. As we work through the phases, we will dive deeper into the micronutrients (think vitamins and minerals) to bring our *total health* full circle.

What Is the Ketogenic Diet?

If it's okay with you, I'm going to start referencing *ketogenic* as *keto* (key-toe) so that we can sound like the cool kids and keep this simple.

I'm currently sitting curled up on my couch writing this section, and I am overly excited to nerd out with you and simplify the things that feel complicated. I invite you to stay with me and take the time to thoroughly digest what you are about to read. Knowledge is power, and the application of that knowledge is power*ful*. I can't wait for you to embrace your inner nerd with me!

As the old saying goes, "Give a man a fish and he will eat for a day; teach a man to fish and he will eat for a lifetime." My goal is not only to teach you how to fish, but to help you become the *fisherman* so that you can do this for yourself and then help others who are struggling. Many weight-loss plans give you just enough information (in exchange for a dollar) to keep you coming back for more. We are done with that mentality. It's time to learn how this works, learn why this works, and put a plan into action.

Knowledge is power, and the application of that knowledge is powerful.

You will quickly learn that the more you begin to understand the science behind the foods you are eating, the easier it will be for you to stick to the plan on the hard days. When you truly comprehend how toxic your former lifestyle habits were to your body, it's easy to see why you aren't where you want to be right now. But don't worry. It will take only a few days to begin this transition to wellness and get you on your way to feeling and looking incredible.

The keto diet is a style of eating that focuses on a higher intake of healthy fats, a moderate intake of protein, and a very low intake of carbs and sugars. If this already sounds complicated, do not fear. I am going to hold your hand as we break this down into a super simple formula.

The fact is what you *eat* will directly impact how you look and feel. Period. End of story. (Okay, not really. We have a lot more ground to cover.)

We have to find the right combination of foods to consume to help us drop the weight, keep it off, and feel amazing during the process. The keto diet is going to help us do just that. The goal is to eat foods we actually enjoy that are simple to make while simultaneously shrinking our waistlines.

> *The fact is what you **eat** will directly impact how you look and feel. Period.*

We are at a really interesting place in the world right now when it comes to diet and fitness. There are a wide variety of diets and approaches to nutrition that fill your Pinterest boards and Instagram feeds, and many of them are backed by success stories and documented with the results of real-life people just like you. But all this information and the seemingly endless options for beginning your weight-loss journey can be paralyzing.

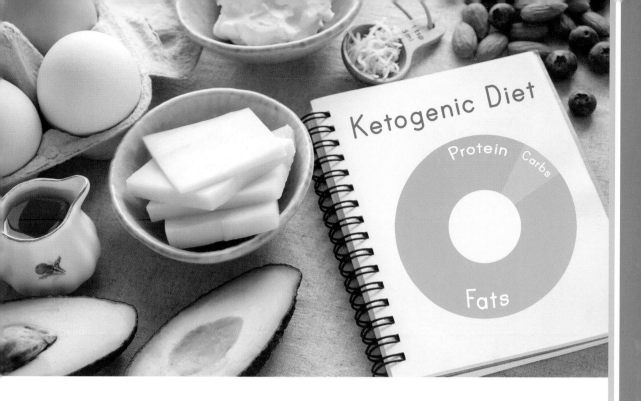

What feels even more confusing is that for every positive article you read about anything, there is an equal and opposite negative article. The information overload available at our fingertips can be overwhelming and prevent most of us from wanting to even start in the first place for fear of doing it wrong.

You've already taken a huge step by reading this book and choosing to take action. I'm going to show you how keto works and *why* it works, and give you a simple approach to getting started in this way of eating. There are many diet styles out there that are just as effective from a weight-loss perspective, but many people find the keto diet to be something they can stick to for the long term because it's awesome! (Just wait until you see my keto pizza! Yeah, I said it: keto *pizza*.)

Before we get into the technical parts of keto, I want to discuss how our body gains energy from the foods we eat.

Food is the fuel that keeps us feeling good and optimizes our metabolism to burn fat. When we eat, our body uses different macronutrients as fuel. Macronutrients (or "macros") can sound like a complex term, but it's actually simple.

Our macros are basically:

- Fat
- Protein
- Carbohydrates

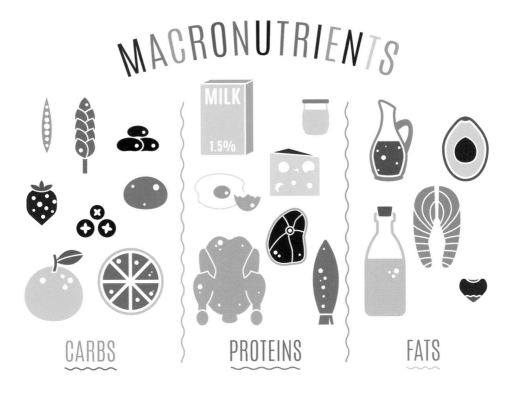

When we take in a moderate to high amount of carbohydrates, our body naturally burns those carbs as fuel to sustain our energy. The reason for that is our body burns through carbohydrates first during the oxidative process because carbohydrates are the quickest and most readily available energy source.

By consuming a moderate to high amount of carbohydrates (as characterized by the "standard American diet"), we are automatically "carb-burners." Being a carb-burner in and of itself is not a bad thing. The problem arises when we take in more carbohydrates than our body needs, which causes our body to store the excess carbohydrates as fat.

When we follow a keto diet, we remove the majority of our carbohydrates, which leaves our body needing fuel. When no fuel is available in the form of carbohydrates, our body becomes a "fat-burner" and uses fats from both our food and our fat stores on our body as fuel. I don't know about you, but there is something about the idea of being a "fat-burner" that really gets me all fired up!

I don't know about you, but there is something about the idea of being a "fat-burner" that really gets me all fired up!

The Sugar Situation

I haven't found a sugar-laden food item yet that I don't love. Put it in front of me, and I have to dig deep to find the willpower to say no. Before I started eating a keto diet, I couldn't stop thinking about sugary foods. My body craved them, and I could have put up a hard argument as to why I *needed* them to survive. When I ate a sugary meal, I felt so happy for about an hour, until it all came crashing down. This would send me straight to the kitchen for more sugar. It was a cycle of cravings I thought I would never overcome.

> *If Carboholics Anonymous was a thing, I would have been the founder.*

When I first *considered* a ketogenic diet, even I thought I was insane. No sugar? Like, at all? Ever? How would I live without sugar?! If Carboholics Anonymous was a thing, I would have been the founder. We would have T-shirts, regular meetings for support, and friendship bracelets from Etsy.

Sugar was the *only* food group I cared about, and the only thing that made me feel like I was halfway sane. I thought, *God, please love the close friends and family in my life because I am about to be downright awful.*

It turned out that it was not *nearly* as challenging as it seemed. Don't get me wrong. Reversing old habits is tough, but I have a feeling that you, my dear, are tougher. Remember, if the carb queen can slay her sugar dragons, so can you.

We will discuss the phases to my keto diet plan later, but when it comes to cutting sugar, there are two ways to approach the start of your sugar restriction: rip off the Band-Aid or taper down slowly. I've always been the all-in type, so the ripping off of Band-Aids was the only thing that made sense to me. However, I have worked with many women who have tapered their carb intake slowly over a period of a few weeks, and they felt it was easier on their mind and body.

No matter which way you choose, the goal is to get your sugar as low as possible and as quickly as possible.

But why is sugar so bad?

Sugar is the most frequently overused and abused carbohydrate. Sugar is tricky because it is naturally very addicting. Research shows us that sugar is *eight times* more addictive than *cocaine*. Most of us have an underlying sugar addiction that we don't even realize is present, and it's not entirely our fault. Sugar is snuck into the vast majority of processed foods that are labeled as "healthy foods." By consuming sugar repeatedly, our body develops a dependency on it. This is why we eventually cave into cravings. Our body becomes dependent on this sweet little molecule and tricks us into thinking we need more and more of it.

RESEARCH SHOWS US THAT SUGAR IS *EIGHT TIMES* MORE ADDICTIVE THAN *COCAINE*.

When we attempt to go from a diet high in sugar to a diet with moderate amounts of sugar, we are simply managing an addiction. You would never tell someone who was addicted to cocaine to use it occasionally because we all know it would be just a matter of time before the problem got out of control again.

But there are deeper problems with sugar than mere addiction, like insulin resistance. When we hear these words, we think this only pertains to diabetes, but insulin resistance reaches far beyond a diabetic condition.

Insulin is a hormone produced by the pancreas when we consume glucose (sugar) in our diet. Insulin is necessary because it helps our cells absorb the glucose we consume and converts it into energy for our body.

New studies are published regularly regarding insulin resistance, as it is something that is becoming more and more recognized in the health field. What we *do* know for sure is that our body can handle only so much sugar, and when we repeatedly eat too much of it, our body develops a resistance.

Insulin resistance is often linked to conditions like:

- Diabetes
- Obesity
- Polycystic ovarian syndrome (PCOS)
- Inflammatory disorders
- Vascular disease
- Metabolic syndrome

Regardless of whether you have an underlying resistance to insulin, there is good news: insulin resistance can be improved through your diet.

EACH PERSON'S BODY IS DIFFERENT.

When we remove the majority of carbohydrates (specifically sugar) from our diet, our body transitions into a fat-burning state called ketosis and begins burning fat as our fuel. This makes us fat-burners rather than carb-burners. When we are in a fat-burning mode, our body not only burns the fat from our food as fuel but also burns the fat stores in our body. We literally turn our extra fat stores into fuel that gives us energy! How cool is that?

Each person's body is different, so the time it takes to fully transition into ketosis can vary from person to person. The body will always deplete its carbohydrates first, so once the carbohydrates are removed from the diet, the body begins a process of glycogen depletion. Once our glycogen stores (carbohydrate stores in liver and muscles) are depleted, our body then turns to a mode of burning fats as fuel. On average, our body will transition into ketosis around days three to five.

But . . . Will Fat Make Me Fat?

After the Industrial Revolution, our culture saw a huge shift in the standard American diet (also known as SAD). Fat became grossly misunderstood, and we began eliminating it from our diet. When these crucial healthy fats were eliminated, carbohydrate intake rose.

Fast-forward to now, and the average American consumes 152 pounds of sugar each year![1] *One hundred and fifty-two pounds!* It's no wonder that disease is on the rise and our waistlines are expanding.

According to the American Heart Institute, we should limit sugar and carbohydrate consumption to 25 grams per day for women and 38 grams per day for men.[2] These recommendations apply to *any* style of diet you choose.

Fat is not the culprit for carrying excess fat, but sugar is.

Research has shown us, through the years, that fat is not the culprit for carrying excess fat, but sugar is.

When low-fat diets became all the rage, we immediately replaced our fat consumption with sugar and processed carbohydrates. Since then, the obesity rate has tripled, along with the prevalence of type 2 diabetes.

The good news? Following a ketogenic diet can reverse many diseases and can heal your body from the inside out. By using fats as fuel, we actually burn all of the fat we consume and do not have to worry about gaining more fat.

How to Recognize Ketosis

Once the carbs are reduced, the big question is: How will you know if you are in ketosis?

I started a keto diet back in early 2015, way before keto was cool. Most people had heard of a low-carb approach, but the vast majority of people had no idea what ketosis was or why I was doing it. There were no special monitors to tell you if you were in ketosis. And I think it was so much better that way. We don't need another number to judge ourselves with and base our progress on. I relied on how I felt mentally and physically to know if I was on the right track.

There are many different ways and tests on the market to determine when you are in ketosis, but the best way is to listen to your body. When we have transitioned into ketosis, our body begins to produce ketones. Ketones are produced by your liver to help your body burn fats as fuel. And once you have fully transitioned, you will begin to feel an abundance of clean energy. You should also notice that any brain fog is gone and that your mental clarity is at an all-time high. Also, as your inflammation begins to decrease, you should experience a noticeable difference in physical swelling.

Once you have fully transitioned, you will begin to feel an abundance of clean energy.

TEST ONCE A DAY, THE SAME TIME EACH DAY.

But if you don't mind the expense and really *need* to know for sure, the best option for ketone testing is a blood ketone monitor. Though it is not 100 percent accurate, it is the most accurate way to detect if your body is producing ketones. When using a blood ketone monitor, be sure to test once a day, the same time each day—approximately one hour after waking. If you test at random times throughout your day, you may get a false positive or false negative.

Here is an excerpt from the Keto-Mojo blood monitor website:

If your primary goal for integrating the ketogenic diet into your life is weight loss, achieving "light nutritional ketosis," or 0.5 mmol/L–1.0 mmol/L, is a good starting point. From there, aim for "optimal ketosis," which is when your ketone levels are between 1.0 mmol/L–3.0 mmol/L. . . .

People who are fasting or eat a much higher fat-to-protein ratio will look to levels in the 3.0 mmol/L–8.0 mmol/L range. But you don't need to go there. The optimal ketosis range is called "optimal" for a reason, and it's exactly where you'll want to be for weight-loss and general health purposes, and you'll get there, in time, if you practice patience and get in the groove of eating a keto diet.[3]

The other alternative to ketone testing is using urine strips. If you have these handy, I recommend throwing them into the trash. (Kidding kind of.) Urine ketone strips are known to be *highly* inaccurate. I don't know about you, but I don't see much point in going through a process that is known to be inaccurate. In addition to inaccuracies, the ketone test strips typically test for only *one* kind of ketone. Since our body produces three different kinds, it is not uncommon for a test strip to be negative because it's only picking up trace amounts of the specific ketone it detects.

If you test your ketones and the results reflect you are not in ketosis, do not let this derail your progress! You *must* develop the ability to trust the process and stay on your path. It is so very tempting to think it isn't working and give up. Remember, you do not have to be in ketosis to lose weight. While it is the overall goal to reach a place where our body is producing ketones (and burning fat as fuel), it is not the end-all-be-all of weight loss.

Remember, you do not have to be in ketosis to lose weight.

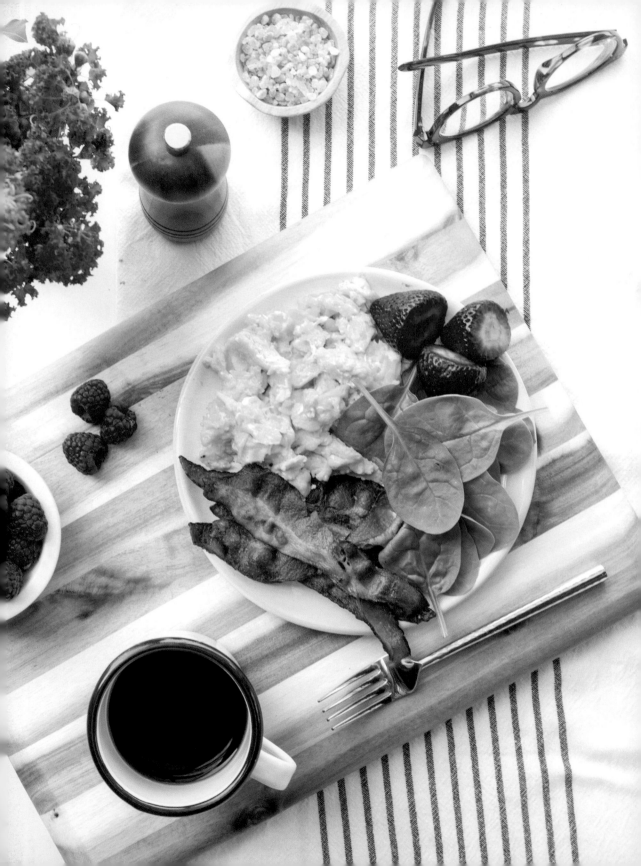

6

THE KETOGENIC PLAN

My approach to the keto lifestyle is a bit different from most traditional keto diets out there, because the focus is on *transitional* wellness. In my own journey, and my experience coaching others, I have found that lasting results are found from taking a stair-step approach and building a foundation of habits that will last a lifetime.

In general, most of us cannot go from overall unhealthy habits to overall super-healthy habits overnight. Even if we can muster up the courage to go all in, most of us will eventually feel overwhelmed and fall back on our old habits. This four-phase approach infuses our mind-set transformation into our diet changes so that we can get off the diet roller coaster and stick to this for life.

I am not interested in providing you with tools to "lose thirty pounds *fast*!" only for you to get frustrated, overwhelmed, and fall off the wagon. In these phases, you will find a gentle transition that will get the scale moving and help you transition to your new healthy lifestyle with ease.

Getting Started

One of my favorite parts of the ketogenic diet is that you can eat virtually anywhere. Whether you are someone who loves to cook or you are a busy executive on the road, this style of dieting will work for you!

And that's the key. For too long, we have tried to make our lifestyle mold to a diet. We have to flip the script and figure out how to make our diet style match our life. It's the only way to stick it out long term.

In the pages that follow, I will provide variations of sample meal plans that will give you exactly what you need to start your keto diet, but there are some tried and true principles that can be applied to your daily life right away. One of the key fundamentals of the ketogenic diet is to break away from dependence on sugars and carbs. That means cutting them off at the source.

The good news is that once we cut off the supply, the cravings will slow down and eventually come to a stop. You will come to a point where food is rarely on your mind (I actually have to remember to eat). This is one of the most freeing feelings . . . no longer being a slave to food.

This is one of the most freeing feelings . . . no longer being a slave to food.

Another principle to keep in mind as you get started is to always take a stair-step approach. On the surface, this can feel challenging. Most of us want to go all in and do everything perfect from day one . . . but that ultimately sets us up to fail. We have years of hardwiring we have to unravel, and it takes time.

Before I started this plan, one of the first ways I

tried to lose weight was to look at the calories I was consuming. Overall, it is true that in order to lose weight we must create a caloric/macro deficit so that our body is burning more calories than it's taking in. So I headed to the Internet and did one of those quizzes to determine how many calories this random website suggested. (I was putting my fate into the hands of someone I didn't know, but they *had* to know more than I did, right?)

My result? Thirteen hundred calories. Sounded good to me!

Overall, I had always been conscious of what kinds of foods I should and should not be eating. Deep down, I think we all are. Broccoli . . . likely on the good list. Cake . . . probably should lay off a bit. So I started this 1,300-calorie plan with the full intention of eating 1,300 calories' worth of nutritious foods.

The problem was I had years of bad habits I continued falling victim to. I was still addicted to sugar. And it's not likely I would go from being a fast-food junkie to a superfood maven overnight. (Have I mentioned that I still hate kale?)

After a few days, my 1,300-calorie diet started to look more like two really big, high-calorie meals. Then I was not eating all day so that I could binge all 1,300 calories at night, which led to falling off the wagon completely. The vicious cycle was becoming worse.

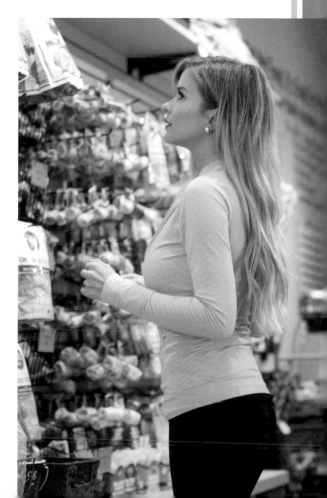

I had to begin changing the way I was looking at meals. Instead of simply counting calories, I began focusing on macronutrients and consuming the proportions of each that work for my body.

In this phase of the plan, we are focusing on hitting macronutrient targets, not just calories. As an example, let's say that two different people decide to follow the 1,300-calorie diet mentioned above to create a caloric deficit and promote weight loss. The first person decides to eat 1,300 calories' worth of cookies each day. The second person decides to eat 1,300 calories' worth of high-fat, low-carb foods. While both may see a drop in the scale (due to being in a caloric deficit), they will each look and feel *very* different. We must come to realize this is about more than just having a goal weight. This is about having a goal life that includes looking and feeling our best.

The vicious cycle was becoming worse.

By adding this level of specificity, we are ensuring that our body gets the macronutrients it is craving to keep our energy and metabolism high while reducing unwanted body fat.

Now that we have covered a high-level overview of the ketogenic diet, I'm excited to dive right into our phased approach.

Phase One

If you are like me, you are coming into this diet eating way more sugars and carbs than you even realize. And that's okay. It's not about who you *were* or what you *did*. It's all about what you are doing about it *now*. You can change . . . just like that.

THE FOCUS OF PHASE ONE IS SIMPLE:

1. Reduce sugar and carbs as much as possible.
2. Increase healthy fats.
3. Drink lots of water.
4. Begin to move your body.

During this phase, we will transition to eating as little sugar and carbs as possible and not worry about any restrictions in other areas (such as tracking, food timing, portion size, etc.).

Phase one is intended for those who have not been dieting or who get a little nervous about starting a new plan. The goal is to keep it as simple as possible and move to phase two when you have mastered phase one.

If you are approaching a keto lifestyle and have previously mastered discipline in your eating habits, then this phase should be skipped, and you can begin with phase two.

During phase one, you should make it a goal not to allow yourself to get too hungry. Keep some nuts handy (I love flavored almonds) and eat a few any time you start to feel hungry (or have cravings). The reason there is no limit to the amount of food we eat in this phase is because when we let our hunger get ahead of us, our head starts doing the talking. Next thing you know, you have convinced yourself to eat sweets when you really only needed a healthy meal.

Reducing Sugar and Carbs

The best way to starve any addiction (like sugar) is to cut it off at the source and go cold turkey. However, not all of us are created equal, and some see more success with a taper-down strategy.

For example, if you are drinking six full-sugar sodas a day, you could plan to taper down by half of a can every three days until you are no longer drinking them. Another example would be to replace your sugary sodas with a sugar-free variety (we will look at sugar replacements a little later).

To start removing sugar and carbs, you can do the following:

- Remove bread and eat sandwiches and burgers on their own; try lettuce wraps or portobello mushrooms in place of the bread.
- Skip the rice and/or beans and replace with veggies.
- Avoid pasta dishes.
- Skip foods that have sugar or flour listed as an ingredient.

Increasing Healthy Fats

When we remove the sugar and carbs from our diet and replace them with healthy fats, this helps ensure we have enough energy to fuel our body. This also helps us keep our skin healthy and our metabolism high.

Here are a few high-fat ideas to raise your healthy fat intake:

- Add one tablespoon of healthy oil when cooking. (See page 159 for ideas.)
- Snack on nuts (I like macadamia nuts and flavored almonds).
- Add half of an avocado to your meals.
- If you eat dairy, add butter, cheese, or heavy whipping cream.

KEEP SOME
NUTS HANDY.

Remember, transitioning to this style of eating takes time. Before you know it, you will be a pro!

A Word on Protein

In this phase, continue eating the amount of protein you normally consume. In phase two, we will tighten down a more specific goal in regard to protein. As we mentioned briefly before, the general layout for each plate is highest in healthy fats, moderate in protein, and lowest in carbohydrates.

Hydration

I know, I know . . . it's important to drink water. (I always roll my eyes when my doctor suggests I should be more hydrated.) But water is serious business when it comes to a ketogenic diet.

When we transition into a state of ketosis, our body naturally depletes itself of its water storage. This is amazing news, because it means we can kiss bloating goodbye! But it also means we make ourselves vulnerable to dehydration.

The term *keto flu* is thrown around pretty loosely and scares people out of trying this style of dieting. It certainly did for me at first. Any diet that has the ability to produce flu-like symptoms doesn't sound like a diet I want to follow.

But the reality is the keto flu is nothing more than dehydration, and it can easily be avoided.

INCREASE

HEALTHY

FATS.

SOME TIPS TO PREVENT DEHYDRATION OR FLU-LIKE SYMPTOMS:

- Aim to drink 70 to 100 ounces of water each day.
- Drink 8 ounces of bone broth.
- Drink electrolyte-enriched water.
- Add additional salt to your food (sodium is an electrolyte).
- Supplement potassium and magnesium.

If at the beginning of this process you are a long way from drinking a gallon of water each day, remember that taking a stair-step approach is always best when building lifelong habits. Start by taking a day to measure how much water you normally drink without making any changes. You'll naturally be tempted to drink more now that you're aware of the importance of hydration during the keto diet, but try your best to get a true sample of your starting point by simply logging your normal water intake. At the end of the day, add up the total ounces of water you consumed and commit to increasing your intake incrementally until you get to the goal. You'll meet your smaller goals along the way—yay!—and find that drinking 70 to 100 ounces of water per day is easier to do than you might have imagined.

Move Your Body

In a later section, we will go into the specifics of moving our bodies, but I want to go ahead and encourage you to get started. Exercise is so crucial to feeling good, both mentally and physically. Even a few minutes of movement is a powerful way to begin, and every minute adds up.

Transitioning to Phase Two

Your goal should be to move to phase two as quickly as you can. However, you should have a good grasp on the current phase before moving forward. Moving too quickly to the next phase can result in relapse (going back to old habits).

There are no rules here. This journey is about you, your mind, and your body. You should stay in this phase for as long as you need to while also making a plan and a goal to push yourself toward the next phase.

Phase Two

In phase two, we will take everything we learned from phase one and kick it up a notch. You will likely spend a good portion of your weight-loss journey in this phase. Phase two is taking the same higher-fat/lower-carb model and adding more structure and specificity.

> # IN ADDITION TO FOCUS POINTS OF PHASE ONE, THE FOCUS OF PHASE TWO CONSISTS OF:
>
> 1. Tracking food intake based on the Daily Macro Chart (see following pages).
> 2. Preplanning your meals.
> 3. Eating on a schedule.
> 4. Exercising thirty minutes each day, five days per week.

Tracking Daily Food Intake

When we are discerning about the specific foods we consume, we ensure we are going to be successful in losing weight and also looking and feeling our best. We do this by stabilizing our blood sugar, giving our body the healthy fats it needs for energy, and eliminating as much processed, sugary foods as possible. Your body will love you for it!

In the beginning, the idea of tracking my foods made me feel like I was in prison. It felt like an unnecessary chore, and I tried to avoid it for as long as possible. But the problem with not tracking is that you are flying blind and have no idea how much you are consuming. Even four years later, I often find myself so surprised at the macros that make up certain foods.

In the following charts, you will find a list of daily macronutrient goals based on your *current* weight and activity level. The goal is to start where you are and taper down as the weight comes off.

DAILY MACRO CHART

Not Active to Lightly Active 1–3 days/week

Current Weight	Fat Goal	Protein Goal	Net Carb Goal	Calorie Range
>300 lb.	130g Fat	80g Protein	<25g Net Carbs	1525–1655 calories
275–299 lb.	125g Fat	75g Protein	<25g Net Carbs	1460–1590 calories
250–274 lb.	120g Fat	73g Protein	<25g Net Carbs	1407–1537 calories
225–249 lb.	115g Fat	68g Protein	<25g Net Carbs	1342–1472 calories
200–224 lb.	110g Fat	65g Protein	<25g Net Carbs	1285–1415 calories
175–199 lb.	105g Fat	63g Protein	<25g Net Carbs	1232–1362 calories
150–174 lb.	100g Fat	60g Protein	<25g Net Carbs	1175–1305 calories
<150 lb.	95g Fat	60g Protein	<25g Net Carbs	1130–1260 calories

Lightly Active to Moderately Active (+10%)

Current Weight	Fat Goal	Protein Goal	Net Carb Goal	Calorie Range
>300 lb.	143g Fat	88g Protein	<25g Net Carbs	1674–1804 calories
275–299 lb.	138g Fat	83g Protein	<25g Net Carbs	1603–1733 calories
250–274 lb.	132g Fat	80g Protein	<25g Net Carbs	1544–1674 calories
225–249 lb.	127g Fat	75g Protein	<25g Net Carbs	1473–1603 calories
200–224 lb.	121g Fat	72g Protein	<25g Net Carbs	1410–1540 calories
175–199 lb.	116g Fat	69g Protein	<25g Net Carbs	1352–1482 calories
150–174 lb.	110g Fat	66g Protein	<25g Net Carbs	1289–1419 calories
<150 lb.	105g Fat	66g Protein	<25g Net Carbs	1240–1370 calories

Moderately Active to Heavily Active (+20%)

Current Weight	Fat Goal	Protein Goal	Net Carb Goal	Calorie Range
>300 lb.	156g Fat	96g Protein	<25g Net Carbs	1823–1953 calories
275–299 lb.	150g Fat	90g Protein	<25g Net Carbs	1745–1875 calories
250–274 lb.	144g Fat	88g Protein	<25g Net Carbs	1681–1811 calories
225–249 lb.	138g Fat	82g Protein	<25g Net Carbs	1603–1733 calories
200–224 lb.	132g Fat	78g Protein	<25g Net Carbs	1535–1665 calories
175–199 lb.	126g Fat	76g Protein	<25g Net Carbs	1471–1601 calories
150–174 lb.	120g Fat	72g Protein	<25g Net Carbs	1403–1533 calories
<150 lb.	114g Fat	72g Protein	<25g Net Carbs	1349–1479 calories

When looking at the charts for your fat and protein target, your goal is to come as close to the numbers listed as possible. It won't always be feasible to hit those numbers exactly, but your aim should be to come within 5 grams above or below.

The goal is to start where you are and taper down as the weight comes off.

The other goal here is to come as close to these targets as consistently as possible. If you have a day or two that you go over or under, it's okay! Just like we don't gain a hundred pounds in one day, missing the mark one day will not totally sabotage your efforts.

To determine your activity level, you should look at the past seven days and decide which category would be most accurate. My hope is that you are moving your body moderately each week, which also means you should be increasing how much you eat.

This can feel backward at first. I mean, less is more, right? Well, not always. Our overall goal is to consume as much as we can while still promoting weight loss. This will keep your metabolism at an all-time high, keep you nourished, and keep you full of the nutrients your body craves.

What Fats Should I Eat?

Hitting your fat target is one of the more challenging goals to conquer in this phase, because for so long we have been taught to stay clear of fats. The fats you consume are going to give you the energy you need to fuel your body.

When you first increase your fat intake, it is normal to feel very full and satisfied. This is a great problem to have, since many diet styles leave you feeling hungry and craving more. For so long, we thought that if we eat less, we will lose more, and that is simply not true. Not taking in enough nutrients will actually slow your metabolism, cause you to retain fat, and leave you drained of energy.

In a later section, you will find some great recipe ideas as well as a shopping list. There are some great suggestions there for you to become a fat-burning machine!

How to Reduce Protein Intake

While many of us struggle to cut carbs, proteins are often the dominant force on the plate, and if you've spent years increasing your protein intake, it's likely going to take some focus to make sure you hit your protein target without getting too much. It's so easy to go over.

Activity Journal

Keep a weekly record of your activity and adjust your macros accordingly.

My biggest recommendation to reduce your protein intake is to simply cut your portion size down by 1 to 2 ounces. If you don't have a food scale, it's not a problem. One ounce is about the size of three dice. Even reducing one ounce of chicken (per meal) will save you around 9 grams of protein.

The Carb Goal

When it comes to carbs, no matter where you are on your weight-loss journey, the target is to stay below 25 grams of net carbs each day.

I cannot stress enough how important this step is. And rest assured, you will not have to track forever. Right now you are keeping a record to make sure you are consuming the right quantities of food so that you can get on your path and lose the weight. Tracking takes time, but it is worth it. If you are going to go through the pain of change, you might as well do it right. Fifty percent effort will never get you greater than a 50 percent result. This time is going to be different.

Each day continue to focus on the food-shifting strategy provided. And throughout the day, I also want you to input all the foods you are eating into a tracking app. Thanks to the availability of smartphones, tracking is so much easier than it used to be. There are many apps that can simplify this process and keep you on track, but MyFitnessPal and Carb Manager are my favorites. (A note on MyFitnessPal: It does not automatically show you net carbs, so be sure to manually subtract any sugar alcohols and dietary fiber, which I'll share more about soon.) Note that it is crucial to always double-check the nutrients listed. Most of the available apps have user-submitted data, which leaves great room for error.

One thing that has always made tracking easier for me is to use the

I WAS SHOCKED AT THE AMOUNT OF SUGARS AND CARBS I WAS TAKING IN . . . EVEN AFTER I HAD PULLED SO MANY OUT!

function to input my own foods. I pick five to six meals that I eat on repeat and load the macro count into the app. That way I can quickly input my foods without much thought.

Now, let me warn you: during your first few days of tracking foods, you will likely be *way* off your target macros. I know I was shocked at the amount of sugars and carbs I was taking in . . . even after I had pulled so many out! Don't let this distract you or deter you. Recording all this information is painting a picture for you to see how close you are to being on the right track. Once you can clearly see what your current intake is, it will be easy for you to begin to make small tweaks to get you closer and closer to your goal.

Tracking is so much easier than it used to be.

At the end of the day, take a look at everything you consumed. How could you have removed some of the carbs and sugars? How could you have added more fat? Once you see how you are tracking, you can start making better choices that lead to success in the following days.

Net Carbs

When following a ketogenic diet, we are going to look at *net* carbs instead of total carbs. To calculate the net carbs, take a look at your nutrition label and take the total carbs and subtract any dietary fiber and sugar alcohol.

The overarching goal of the ketogenic diet is to keep our blood sugar consistently stable and not to create an insulin spike. We do this by drastically reducing our carb intake compared to a standard diet.

The reason we do not factor in sugar alcohols and dietary fiber is that these types of carbohydrates do not have a direct impact on our blood sugar and insulin levels.

Even though sugar alcohols do not negatively impact our blood sugar, you should take in as little sugar alcohol as possible. When you begin the ketogenic way of eating, you may lean more heavily on sugar alcohols to kill your sweet tooth, and that's okay! We just want to be sure to come up with a transition plan to slowly taper this down, so you are not taking in large amounts of sugar alcohols on a consistent basis.

Later, we will fully dive into how we are going to take these macros and apply them to real life!

Preplanning Meals

You know what they say: "If you fail to plan, you plan to fail." Even though that quote has been super overused, I have never found that statement to be inaccurate in any scenario. For so many years, we have relied on our emotions to tell us what we should and should not eat. Our emotions are all over the place and cannot be trusted to guide us in these decisions. Remember, the key is to do the *right* thing, despite how you *feel*. When you plan ahead, it's easier to make the right choices.

Remember, the key is to do the right thing, despite how you feel.

Each night before bed, I want you to pull out the ole tracker and plan the following day. You can also use a food-tracking journal to record your daily intake.

When I map out my meals, I like to leave myself a little wiggle room for the occasional Starbucks coffee. (Can I get an *amen*?) One thing I find to be helpful is to take the total macros and divide them by the number of meals I plan on eating so that I can get a per-meal average to shoot for.

One of the biggest struggles I have seen with people trying a keto-genic lifestyle is going over on protein macros. This is likely due to how we've been conditioned as a society to believe that protein should take up the majority of our plate. However, we do not need nearly as much protein as we have been led to believe, and consuming too much can be hard on our kidneys. In addition, high amounts of protein can actually be converted to glucose by the liver through a process called gluconeogen-esis. You may find you need to decrease the amount of protein you have planned. If so, simply cut down your normal serving size by one to two ounces. That will save you big-time by the end of the day.

As you log your foods, compare the total macros from the app to the total macros in the macro chart. If you aren't within 5 grams of your total target, you'll need to make some adjustments. I find adding snacks can help me in the places where I'm falling short.

Eating on a Schedule

In this phase of the plan, your goal is to map out a schedule that works for you and to follow it as consistently as possible. Life happens, and we can't always keep to our plans exactly as they are laid out, but the goal is to build in some consistency to our eating plan.

For this phase, I suggest eating three medium-size meals and one to two snacks each day. It is key to never let your hunger get ahead of you, which requires you to add a bit of structure to your day. Because fats are very satisfying, sometimes we don't really feel hungry at our scheduled eating time and then our hunger comes on very rapidly later in the day.

When I started in this phase, my eating plan looked like this:

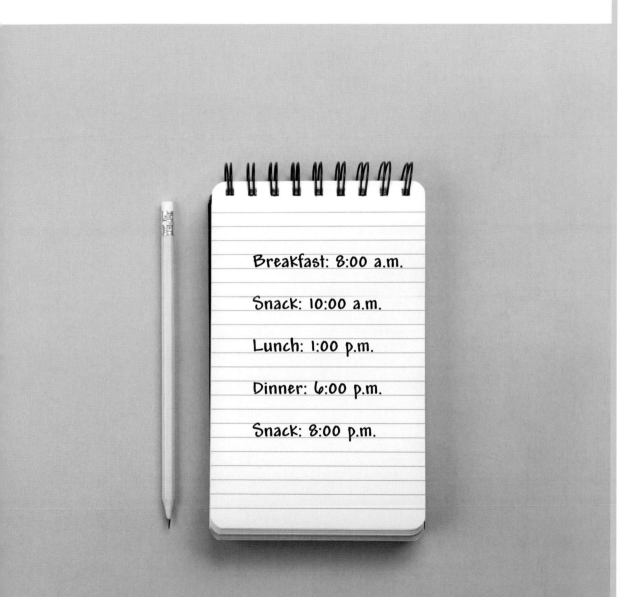

Breakfast: 8:00 a.m.

Snack: 10:00 a.m.

Lunch: 1:00 p.m.

Dinner: 6:00 p.m.

Snack: 8:00 p.m.

MEAL-PLANNING EXERCISE

Now is a great time to put this into practice. Pull out your pen and paper, and create a plan for your new diet style. A few things to consider:

- Do you need a different plan on the weekends due to schedule changes?
- Are certain days more difficult due to work meetings?
- Are you a night snacker who needs to build in the last meal at night?

Once you have your plan mapped out, I suggest keeping it somewhere handy, like in the kitchen, to remind you on a regular basis of your new eating schedule. Before you know it, this schedule will become more like second nature to you as you put the habits into place.

You'll notice I was eating every few hours. I built in my last snack in the evening because I am a habitual nighttime snacker. If you tell me I am not allowed to eat past a certain time, I will certainly eat past that time. I listened to what I know about my body and my habits and found an eating plan that worked.

If you tell me I am not allowed to eat past a certain time, I will certainly eat past that time.

Exercise

In this phase, make it a goal to work up to moving your body for thirty minutes each day, five days a week. (Extra credit, if you do more than that!) Even though this section is dedicated to the keto diet, it's important to me to continue to encourage you to start moving your body more and more.

Exercise isn't something I love, but I know how powerful it is—not only from a physical or weight-loss standpoint, but from a mind-set standpoint as well. This is a great time to take a peek at the workouts in this book (see Part 3) or to find a fun workout class in your area you can commit to.

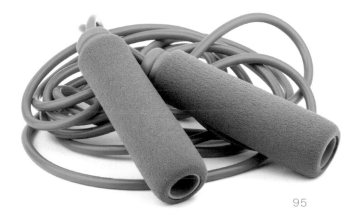

Phase Three

Phase three is going to be super fun for you if you love diving into the details. This phase is very similar to phase two, but we are focusing on the *quality* of our foods and not just the *quantity*.

This transition to wellness is key to optimal health. As we discussed earlier, most of us don't go from eating junk all day to suddenly being the perfect picture of health overnight. Even if we are capable of doing that, it usually isn't sustainable for the long run—which is exactly what this plan is going to help us overcome. Phase two foods aren't bad, but we should always make it a goal to continue to level up our health in all ways as we continue this journey.

To be clear, I lost all of my weight in phase two.

To be clear, I lost *all* of my weight in phase two. You do not have to move to phase three to be successful in weight loss. However, even though I had lost the weight, I didn't feel my health was at the top level that it could have been. When I forged the deep waters of understanding micronutrients (vitamins and minerals) as well as food quality, I saw massive changes. My energy skyrocketed (when I thought it was already great), my skin became bright and glowy, and my hair and nails started growing stronger and thicker.

In my years of being a health coach, I have used phase three as a "thirty-day challenge" many times, and it has taken my clients' weight loss, and their overall health, to a new level. This is a wonderful phase if you have hit a plateau and need to shake it up.

I will warn you: we are going to dive deeper into some nutritional topics. Please don't let it overwhelm you. I feel so strongly that the more we truly understand what we are eating, the greater our opportunity to stick to the plan. It's really hard to go back to eating unhealthy food when you know what's going on beneath the surface.

For this phase, we are following the same plan as phase two, but we are going to talk more specifically about how to change up our plates to recharge our body.

PHASE THREE FOCUS:

1. Eating more nutrient-dense, high-quality foods
2. Tracking daily food intake based on macro chart provided
3. Preplanning your meals
4. Eating on a schedule (with optional intermittent fasting)
5. Exercising thirty minutes a day, five days per week

For this phase we are following the same macronutrient structure as phase two (see page 85). I am so excited to start diving into micronutrients with you as well.

Let's Talk About Fats

During my time in phase two, the vast majority of my fat intake came from dairy (I love all of the cheese). I was slathering everything in butter, drinking all things with heavy whipping cream, and loved anything with cream cheese as the main ingredient. While we will discuss dairy in a later section, I want to change our focus here to where we should get our fats from.

Phase three healthy fat sources:

- Oils, such as coconut oil, avocado oil, sesame oil, and olive oil
- Fatty cuts of organic meat and wild-caught fish
- AVOCADOS! (Sorry, I get excited.)
- Nuts, such as macadamia nuts, almonds, pecans, and pistachios

These are wonderful sources of healthier fat options your body will love. You don't have to immediately make the switch, but make a goal to start filling your plate with more and more of these types of fats, and less and less dairy and mayo.

Keto and Cholesterol

I want to share my personal cholesterol experience.

While we are here, I want to touch on the subject of cholesterol. I am not a cardiologist and would never replace your doctor's advice. However, I discovered I had a lot of misunderstanding about food's role in my cholesterol levels.

First, I want to share my personal cholesterol experience. I have had high familial cholesterol since I was very young. *Familial hypercholesterolemia* is caused by a mutation in the gene for LDL (bad) cholesterol. My level was so high, in fact, that I was actually a special case study at

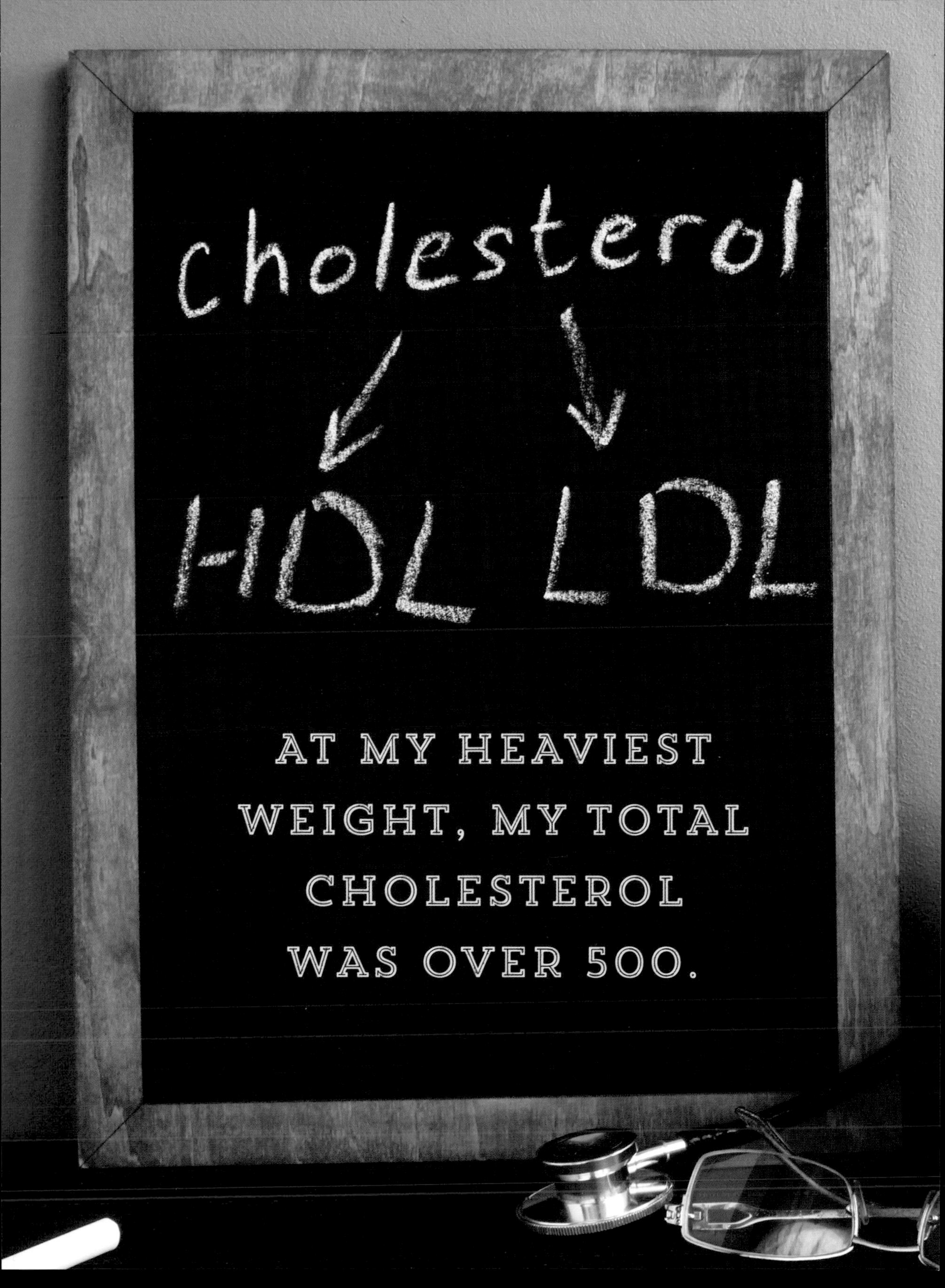

AT MY HEAVIEST WEIGHT, MY TOTAL CHOLESTEROL WAS OVER 500.

Scottish Rite Hospital in second grade. Throughout my entire life, doctors have placed me on low-fat, high-carb diets as a result, and my cholesterol levels kept getting worse and worse. I've been told, more times than I can count, that if I eat too much fat, I will die of a heart attack at a young age. As an added bonus, I am intolerant to all cholesterol-lowering prescription medication. The situation felt hopeless.

> *I didn't realize all of the sugars and carbs I had been eating were actually the drivers behind my cholesterol—not the fats I was consuming.*

At my heaviest weight, my total cholesterol was over 500. It is unlikely you will meet many people with cholesterol *that* high. I'm sure you can imagine the concept of eating a high-fat diet was a little concerning to me, but I was so desperate to lose this weight. My initial plan was to follow the scary high-fat diet until I reached my goal weight; then I would go back to a low-fat diet.

But then the craziest thing happened. Two years into this diet, my bad cholesterol dropped lower than it had ever been in my entire life. And my good cholesterol went up.

So, what gives?

I decided to research this topic. It made no sense to me. I thought fat made us fat! I thought fat gave us high cholesterol. How could my cholesterol possibly be at an all-time low after eating a high-fat diet for so long?

I started researching and found two books by Jimmy Moore with Eric C. Westman, MD, called *Cholesterol Clarity* and *Keto Clarity*, and what I learned was eye-opening.

I won't get into an in-depth science lesson here, but I do want to urge you to pick up these books and begin to understand the science behind fats. I didn't realize all of the sugars and carbs I had been eating were actually the drivers behind my cholesterol—not the fats I was consuming.

Four years into a ketogenic plan, my doctor is 100 percent on board with my continuing, as my heart health has never been better.

Protein Sources

Up until now, we have been eating any protein sources so long as they fit our daily macro goals. For this phase, we have two goals: increase the consumption of organic, grass-fed meats and wild-caught fish, and decrease the consumption of highly processed meats.

Quality meats to increase:	Processed meats to decrease:
Organic, grass-fed chicken	Bacon (unless nitrate-free)
Organic, grass-fed beef	Lunch meats (unless nitrate-free)
Organic, free-range eggs	Sausage
Wild-caught salmon	Hot dogs

The more I learned about meat quality, the more disgusted I became. I had no idea what I was putting into my body by grabbing the cheapest option at the store. After switching to organic meats and wild-caught fish, I immediately noticed a difference in how I felt—and how food tasted.

The more I learned about meat quality, the more disgusted I became.

Organic meat is preferred for a few reasons:

- Higher vitamin and nutrient density
- Less pesticides used (if any)
- Less antibiotics used (if any)
- No added hormones

Talk about getting more bang for your bite! Simple switches like organic versus nonorganic can help you take your nutrient health to the next level.

Processed Meats

There really isn't a clear-cut definition on what qualifies something as a processed meat. A million Internet searches will never provide a consensus. However, across the board, experts agree that nitrates are one of the main ingredients to eliminate.

Carb Sources

This is where the real fun begins! For phase three, your main focus is to start sourcing the majority of your daily carb intake from fruits, veggies, and nuts. In addition, we will dive deeper into which sugar replacements are best.

Up until now, you may have been getting a lot of your carbs from packaged foods, artificial sweeteners, and low-carb desserts. While all of that is okay in small amounts, the goal is to start packing our carb intake with foods that are full of vitamins and minerals, such as fruits and veggies.

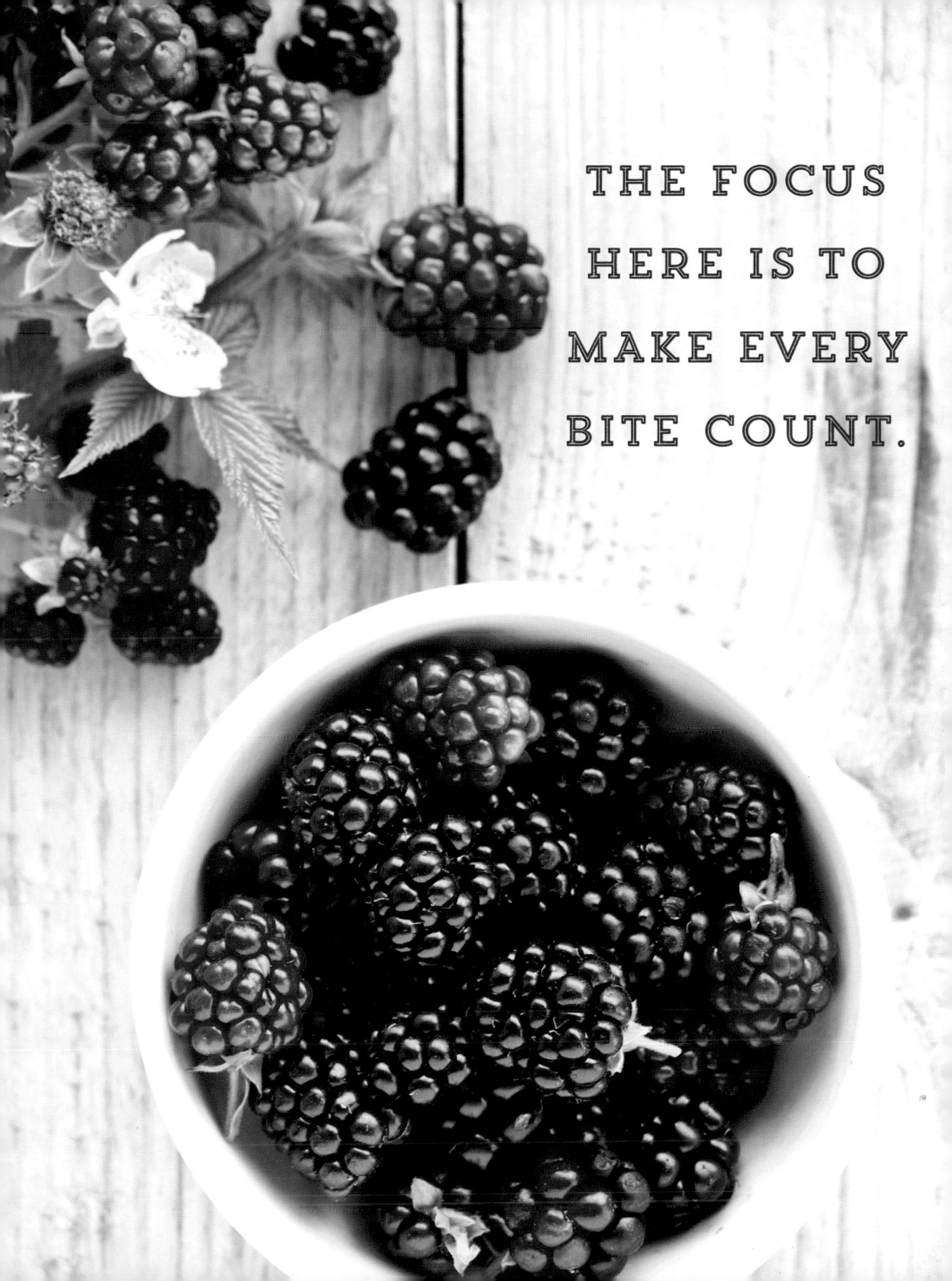

THE FOCUS
HERE IS TO
MAKE EVERY
BITE COUNT.

Carbs to increase in phase three:

- Low-sugar fruits, such as raspberries, blackberries, strawberries, and blueberries
- Green vegetables, such as broccoli, asparagus, green beans, arugula, and spinach
- Colorful veggies, such as bell peppers and spaghetti squash

Carbs to reduce in phase three:

- Low-carb tortillas
- Packaged foods
- Low-carb ice creams

Again, the focus here is to make every bite count. When we source our carb intake from fruits and veggies, we are flooding our body with the vitamins and minerals it needs to make us feel great.

Sugar Replacements

We know we have to kick the real stuff to the curb. But most of us are left with a nagging sweet tooth and still want to be able to sweeten things like drinks and desserts.

I have found that the sooner you can cut the sweet treats, the sooner you abolish all sugar cravings. Often, keto desserts can actually serve as a trigger to crave real sugar. Test this process for yourself to decide whether you can eat low-carb dessert recipes without them becoming a trigger for cravings. In my recipe section, you will notice that I have a few dessert recipes, but I have not included many for this reason.

To understand why some sugar alternatives are better than others, we first need a basic understanding of the glycemic index. The glycemic index is a scale from 1 to 100 that measures the impact certain foods have on your blood sugar. On this scale, sweeteners at 0 would have no impact on blood sugar and sweeteners at 100 would have a full blood sugar spike.

When we are following a ketogenic diet, we want to prevent any spikes in blood sugar so that we maintain a stable and steady blood glucose level at all times. When we eat foods that are too high on the glycemic index, we create a spike in our blood sugar that ultimately knocks us out of ketosis and turns us back into a carb-burner.

If you get knocked out of ketosis at any point, it's no big deal. This can happen after eating a cheat meal. The key is to get right back on track. While it can take a few days to fully transition back into a state of ketosis (where your liver is producing ketones), cheating doesn't have to derail your weight-loss progress.

> *The sooner you can cut the sweet treats, the sooner you abolish all sugar cravings.*

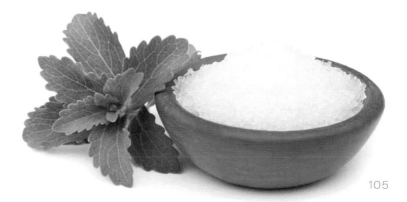

GLYCEMIC INDEX FOR SWEETENERS

Below is a list to show you where sweeteners fall within the glycemic index. This also includes sugar alcohols, which are common forms of sugar replacements. This chart does not contain all sugar substitutes. If you are ever unsure about a sugar substitute that is not listed, I highly suggest researching online.

Sugar: 100

Xylitol: 12

Sorbitol: 4

Stevia: 0

Sucralose: 0

Monk Fruit: 0

Erythritol: 0

When it comes to keto sweeteners, it's important to listen to your body. Some sweeteners can cause gas and bloating while others can cause you to plateau in your weight loss. Everyone's body processes these sweeteners differently, so it's important to determine their impact on you. If you suspect a sweetener may be the culprit of a plateau, I would suggest eliminating it completely for ten days and monitoring how your body feels, as well as the impact on the scale.

Some brands of sweeteners such as Stevia in the Raw and Splenda have an added bulking agent called maltodextrin that is much higher on the glycemic index and can cause stalls. For stevia, always be sure that you check the label and that the only ingredient is stevia. I recommend skipping Splenda altogether.

HERE ARE A FEW FUN FACTS FROM HEALTHLINE:

- Humans are the only species that consume another mammal's milk.
- Seventy-five percent of the world is lactose intolerant.
- Dairy is linked to an increased risk of acne.
- Dairy has been linked to an increased risk of certain cancers.[1]

My favorite sweeteners are stevia and erythritol. Despite their funny-sounding names, both are actually natural sugar replacements and are not chemically made.

Dairy

The consumption of dairy products is a highly debated topic, and it comes down to your own personal experience with reducing or eliminating it completely.

Eliminating dairy isn't like eliminating sugar. You aren't addicted to dairy; you just *like* it. I began the process of going dairy-free after understanding more about how dairy impacts digestion.

I had no idea I was lactose intolerant until I removed dairy from my diet. For years, I have been plagued with chronic allergies, digestive problems, acne, and dull skin. After reading more on the impact of dairy, I decided to eliminate it from my diet.

When eliminating (or reducing) dairy intake, it is important to note that it may take upward of thirty days to notice a significant impact. After my first thirty days of being dairy-free, my allergies cleared up, my asthma disappeared, my skin became clear and bright, and I no longer suffered from the digestive issues that have given me trouble for years.

Additionally, in my coaching experience, I have almost always found that reducing dairy resulted in greater weekly weight loss for my clients. If you don't want to give up dairy completely, I would encourage you to try and eliminate it where you can.

In the shopping list section, you will find lots of great dairy alternatives. Honestly, I have actually come to prefer them over the real thing.

Intermittent Fasting

A huge topic in the ketogenic world is intermittent fasting. Initially, I was turned off to this pattern of eating. I felt like fasting was a form of starvation—aka punishment. However, the more I heard about it, the more I researched and studied it, and eventually, I gave intermittent fasting a try. Now I am a huge advocate for having fasting periods each day and will walk you through exactly what that looks like.

Intermittent fasting (IF) is a pattern of eating where you have a longer fasting window (where no food is consumed) and a shorter eating window (where all macros are consumed).

We all fast every day. That's why the first meal of the day is called "break-fast." We are literally breaking the fast. Most of us naturally fast each day for ten to twelve hours between our last meal and breakfast while we are sleeping. (I'll admit I was approximately thirty years old when I came to this shocking realization, but I digress.)

When following an intermittent fasting plan, we are extending that fast to sixteen hours each day.

Intermittent fasting has a *ton* of benefits that include:

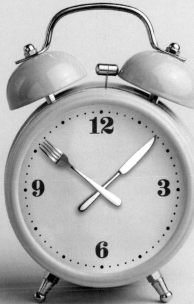

- Increased weight loss
- Gut health and gut repair
- Increased mental clarity and concentration
- Lowered blood sugar
- Lowered cholesterol
- Improvement in fat burning

A typical intermittent fasting window is where you aim to eat all of your macros within an eight-hour period and abstain from food for a sixteen-hour window. During your fasting window, you can consume any beverages that are 5 calories or less. For example, you can drink black coffee, water, or unsweetened tea.

I highly recommend waiting to start an intermittent fasting plan until you have followed the keto plan for at least a full week because you want to allow your body time to begin regulating your blood sugar on its own.

When you first start, I would take a stair-step approach. First, decide what your eight-hour eating window will be. Once your start time has been decided, slowly start eating later and later in the day until you are beginning at your goal time each day. If you normally eat breakfast around 7:00 A.M., I would slowly move your start time back by thirty minutes each day.

I have actually experienced increased mental clarity and energy during the times I am not eating.

A common eating window I have seen is from 10:00 A.M. until 6:00 P.M., which means all meals are consumed during this time. From 7:00 P.M. until 10:00 A.M. the next day, no food is consumed.

Since I am a night owl, my eating window is a little later—typically from 2:00 P.M. to 10:00 P.M. each day. I was initially concerned that not eating before 2:00 P.M. would leave me feeling hungry, tired, and groggy, but I have found the opposite to be true. Once my body adapted to my intermittent fasting period, I have actually experienced *increased* mental clarity and energy during the times I am not eating.

Again, the key is to eat *all* of your macros during this window—and to determine which window works best for you and your schedule. We are simply changing the pattern in which we consume our foods.

For anyone who is recovering (or has recovered) from any form of an eating disorder, use extreme caution when attempting intermittent fasting. In my own journey, I felt I was becoming a bit obsessive about my food intake as I tried to get all of my meals in during a shortened eating window. If at any point you begin to feel you are hyper-focusing on food, I would refrain from intermittent fasting and follow your normal eating pattern.

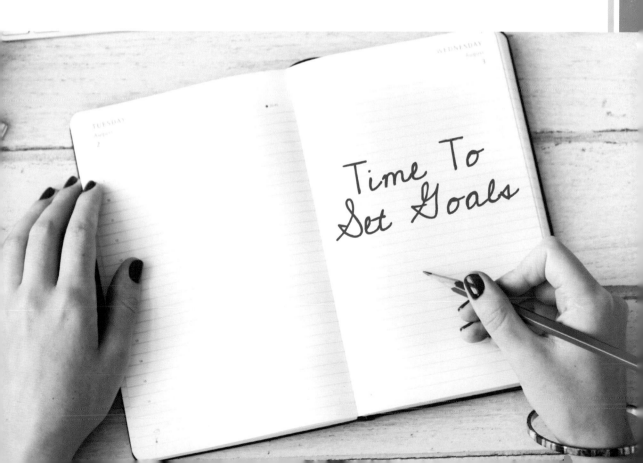

A huge part of overcoming eating disorders is freeing ourselves from the obsessions created around food. For many, intermittent fasting quickly begins to feel like an easy transition. This is not meant to make you feel deprived in any way; it is simply modifying the times when you are consuming your meals.

Small changes make a big impact.

Phase three is a wonderful time for you to challenge yourself and truly embrace your health journey. You may start by incorporating more fruits and veggies or swapping your normal meat for grass-fed, organic meat. As always, making the transition to phase three does not have to be done overnight. Small changes make a big impact in the end, and a stair-step approach is always the best way to build your new habits.

Phase Four

Phase four is #goals. Freedom from food. No, seriously! This is the ultimate place to be. Phase four is all about taking the habits and disciplines we have learned along the way and living life without the chains we carried for so long. This phase is all about freedom to tune in to what your body needs and nourishing it with foods that make you feel good.

Phase four is intended to be followed after you have hit your goal weight—or have come reasonably close. You can also opt to enter phase four if you need a little mental break from tracking your foods in the other phases and want a bit of breathing space from the plan. Remember, taking a short break from following the plan is not the same as ditching it altogether and going back to old, unhealthy habits.

For me, phase four came a couple of years after I hit my goal weight. Even though I was at my goal, I wasn't as focused on healthy and nutritious foods as I should have been. I was still eating a lot of dairy and packaged foods, and although I felt good, I wanted to feel *great*. Once I started focusing on the foods from phase three that nourish my body, I felt better than ever. Now I enjoy a life where I eat healthy foods, I don't have to track every bite, and I focus on how I look and feel mentally, physically, and spiritually.

In this phase, our overall macronutrient balance is the same: a diet highest in healthy fats, moderate in protein, and very low in carbs. However, instead of tracking every bite, we will focus on eating when we are hungry and stopping when we are full.

> *Although I felt good, I wanted to feel great.*

Intuitive Eating

This is a huge buzz phrase in the diet community, particularly around fitness gurus. I love the overall concept of eating based on listening to your body, but it's definitely only appropriate once the foundation from the first three phases has been locked in. If you had asked me to listen to my body when I was first starting, I would have "listened" straight to the donut shop!

Before we break our unhealthy connection to food, the signals our body sends us are confusing. Sugar addiction tricks us into thinking we need things we don't, and cravings convince us we're hungry when we are not. After following the progression from phase one to phase three, we

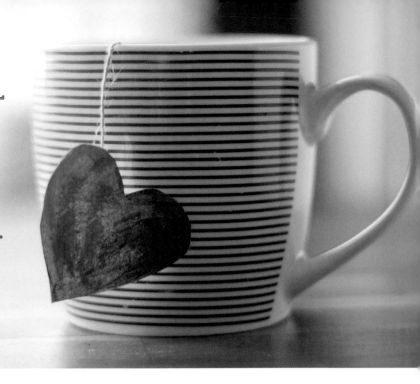

I CAN FILL UP MY BODY'S PHYSICAL LOVE CUP.

have begun to master the mind-set behind our unhealthy habits, healed our triggers, and developed discipline to last a lifetime.

So, what exactly *is* intuitive eating? Intuitive eating is learning to lean in and listen to what your body is telling you it needs. As an example, craving sour foods (like vinegar), can actually be a signal that the liver is not functioning optimally. When we crave salt, it can be a sign of dehydration. Our body has such incredible ways to show us what it needs, and we have to learn to listen to the cues it gives us.

Intuitive eating is also about releasing the feelings of guilt that are associated with certain foods. When we feed our body what it needs, we honor our body. This is a huge step in the way of self-love to find out exactly what our body needs and to give it more of those things.

One of my staple meals is a simple piece of salmon and some avocado with salt on top. I don't particularly love how this meal *tastes*, but after I eat it, I feel so satisfied and my energy is incredible. I know that when I'm a little low on energy, I can fill up my body's physical love cup with a meal that nourishes me.

When we feed our body what it needs, we honor our body.

In this phase of our plan, we still want to stay away from foods we know do not provide us the macro- and micronutrients we need. Intuitive eating is not about throwing healthy habits out the window but experiencing the freedom to eat the foods you feel you need to eat when your body tells you it needs them.

Intuitive eating is a learned skill and won't be mastered overnight. However, when transitioning from a structured plan to a less structured plan, you will still have months' worth of daily habits that will keep you where you desire to be.

A great example would be if you are in this phase and decide to start intensifying your workouts. When we have an increase in energy expenditure through exercise, our body will naturally crave more food and nutrients. You will likely feel a bit hungrier with the addition of a new workout plan, so you are going to let yourself eat until you are not hungry anymore.

Monitoring Weight Gain

Phase four is centered around freedom, and part of that freedom is not being so emotionally tied to a number on the scale. In this phase we want to embrace our bodies and fuel them with the right foods and exercise them with workouts that boost our health.

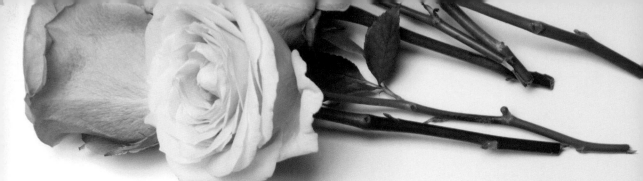

Breakfast (12:00 P.M.): Eggs and Avocado. Lots of energy. Good focus.

Snack (2:00 P.M.): Shrimp Ceviche. Low energy. Brain fog.

Lunch (4:00 P.M.): Bunless Burger Bowl. Medium energy. Good focus.

Dinner (6:00 P.M.): Cashew Crack Slaw. Lower energy. Good focus.

Snack (8:00 P.M.): Protein shake. Medium energy. Low focus.

Every few days, I'll take a quick step on the scale to see where I am. I learned to let go of the weight-gain fear and use it as a number to simply guide me. If it has gone up, I know I may be taking in a bit more food than I need. If it has gone down (unintentionally), I know I need to focus on increasing my food intake to maintain my target weight for my body.

Everyone has a different target weight. I'm tired of the charts in my search engine that tell me what the number on the scale should say. My goal weight is not a number; it's a feeling. I know I am where I want to be based on how my clothes fit, how I feel, and my overall physique. If I am looking too lean, I increase my calories and macros as well as my strength training. If I am getting thick in some areas, I decrease my calories and macros and increase cardio exercise. It's about balance and being in tune with my body.

Getting Started with Intuitive Eating

For this phase, continue following the same eating pattern you have been following up until this point, including how often and the types of foods you eat.

Instead of using a tracking app (or journaling) to track your specific macros, I suggest writing down the meals you ate. Pay close attention to your body after finishing a meal and observe how the food made you feel.

In my example on the opposite page, you will notice that after my shrimp ceviche I had low energy. That is likely because while shrimp ceviche is low in carbs, it is also lower in healthy fats, and it didn't give my body enough energy. Knowing this, I can opt to add some macadamia nuts or healthy oils with my meal next time and then monitor how the added fats made me feel.

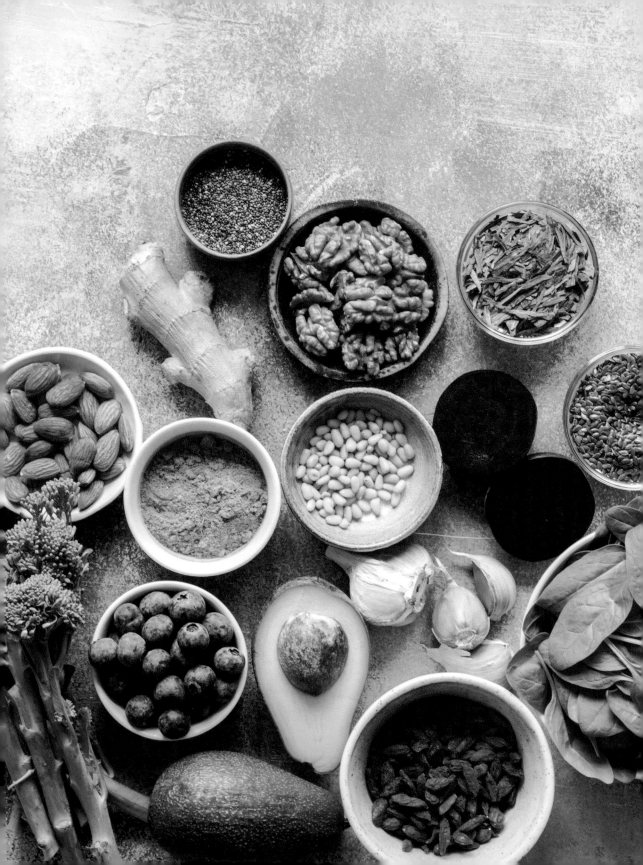

KETO FOR VEGETARIANS
AND VEGANS

One of my favorite parts about the ketogenic style of eating
is that you can follow it despite any food limitations or preferences.
Because traditional keto has a lower protein requirement than other diet
styles, it's easily attainable for both vegans and vegetarians. Overall, following a keto diet while also being a vegan or vegetarian is a great choice.
In Chapter 12, I have provided a sample meal plan so that you can get an
overall view of what your meals should look like.

In my experience, there are three reasons someone chooses a vegan
or vegetarian lifestyle: for personal reasons, for health reasons, or because
they hope it will help them achieve greater weight loss.

The problem for my carb-loving vegan and vegetarian friends is that a
lot of us fall into the trap of eating lots of sugars and carbs and not enough

fruits and vegetables. In most cases (aside from animal-rights activists), this defeats the whole purpose of becoming a vegan or a vegetarian in the first place!

In this section, we are going to focus on the plant-based sources you *should* eat, how to incorporate healthy fats, and how to ensure you're taking in the nutrients you need to look and feel your best.

Healthy Fat Options

Aside from avocados (my favorite), most fruits and vegetables that are low-sugar are not naturally high in healthy fats. A great option is to sauté your favorite vegetables in oils to make them packed with both healthy fats and nutrients.

Here are some great fat options:

- Oils: coconut oil, avocado oil, olive oil, walnut oil, sesame oil, cocoa butter, and grass-fed ghee
- Nuts and seeds: macadamia nuts, almonds, flavored almonds (watch for hidden sugars), walnuts, pecans, pistachios, cashews, pine nuts, Brazil nuts, sunflower seeds, hemp heart seeds, and chia seeds
- Nut butters (check label for added sugar): peanut butter, almond butter, cashew butter, cacao butter, sunflower seed butter, and macadamia nut butter

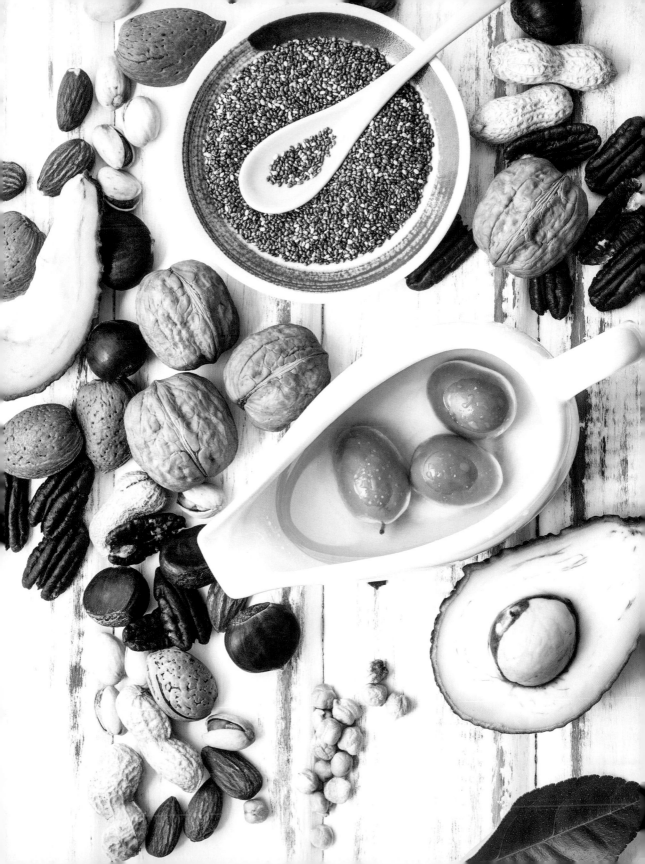

Protein Options

Below are some great vegetarian and vegan options to hit the moderate protein requirement for the keto diet:

- Edamame: 1 cup = 17 protein grams
- Plant-based protein powder: 2 scoops = 20 protein grams (my favorite is OWYN brand)
- Ripple milk (almond): 1 cup = 8 protein grams
- Beyond Meat Burger (vegan): 1 patty = 20 protein grams
- Seitan: 3 ounces = 21 protein grams
- Chia seeds: 1 ounce = 4 protein grams

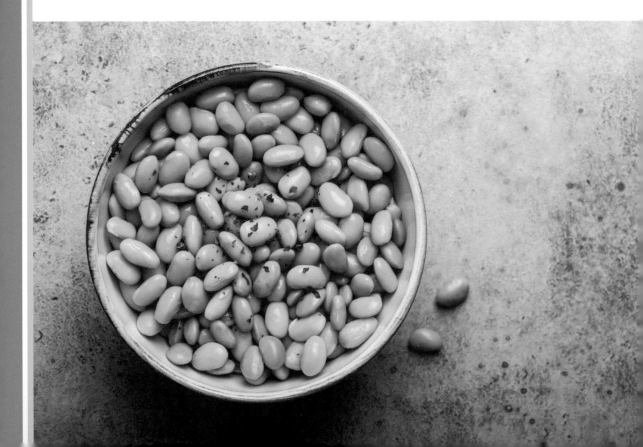

Low-Carb Fruits and Veggies

To keep our overall carb intake to a minimum, focus on fruits and veggies lowest in net carbs. This list is a great starting place!

Veggies

Artichokes

Asparagus

Avocados

Bell peppers

Broccoli

Brussels sprouts

Cabbage

Cauliflower

Celery

Cilantro

Cucumbers

Dark leafy greens: kale, mustard greens, and collard greens

Eggplant

Garlic

Green beans

Lettuce (all kinds)

Mushrooms

Onions

Radishes

Sauerkraut

Scallions and chives

Spaghetti squash

Spinach and chard

Summer squash

Tomatoes

Zucchini

Fruits

Blackberries

Blueberries

Lemons

Limes

Raspberries

Strawberries

Dairy Swaps

Many standard keto recipes call for dairy (in the form of cheese, butter, or heavy whipping cream), but there are several simple swaps. Below are some great dairy alternatives.

Milk

Unsweetened coconut milk

Unsweetened cashew milk

Unsweetened almond milk

Heavy Cream

Make coconut cream by placing a can of coconut milk in the fridge overnight and scooping out the cream off the top.

Butter

Coconut oil

Vegan butter (my favorite is Earth Balance)

Cheese

Vegan cheese or cream cheese (my favorite cheese substitute brands are Kite Hill, Daiya, and Vegan Gourmet).

Eggs

When a recipe calls for eggs, flaxseeds are a great binder. One tablespoon of finely ground flax seed combined with 3 tablespoons of water replaces one egg.

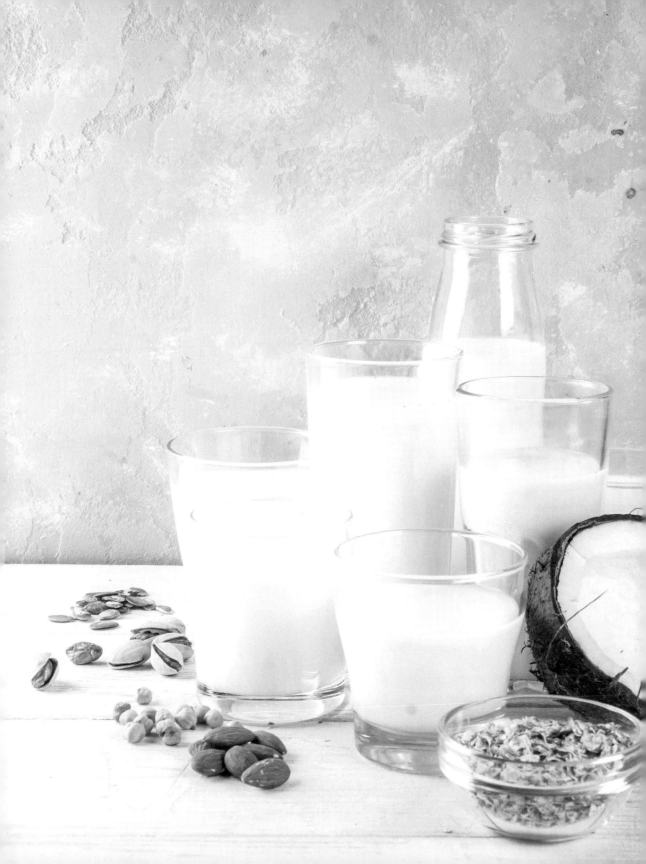

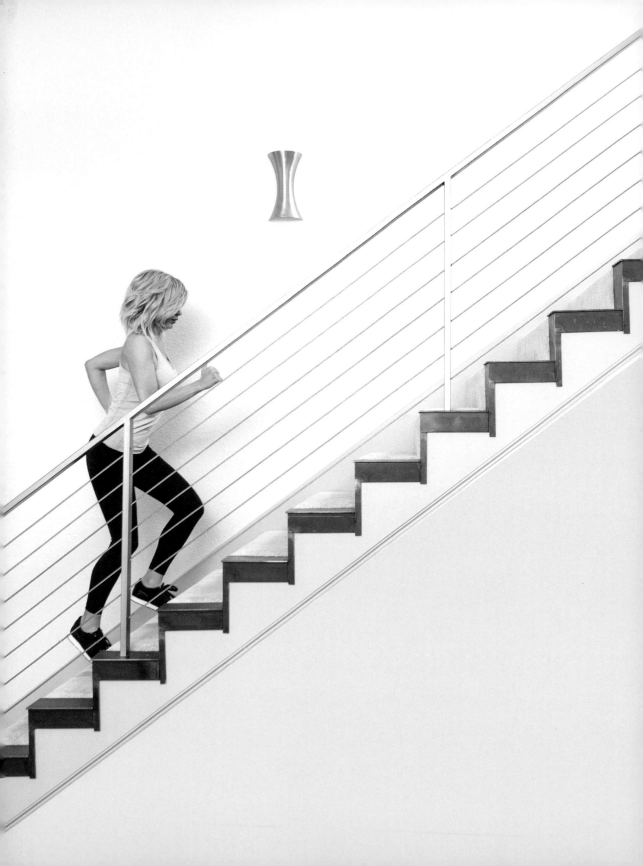

FREQUENTLY
ASKED QUESTIONS

After reviewing a lot of the common questions that I receive on a day-to-day basis, I wanted to devote some time to giving you answers you may be looking for along the way.

What If I Am Stalled?

First, let's define what a true stall is in association with the ketogenic diet. A stall is defined as a period of ten or more days of consistently following the plan where no weight loss occurs. I know, I know, we want to see results overnight. However, we didn't gain weight overnight, and weight loss does not work any differently.

If you have been following the plan and are not seeing results, then it's time to take a look at how much you are consuming. During my weight loss, I played around with my fat macros by increasing (or decreasing) them by 10 percent. In almost all cases, I saw an immediate change in weight.

Remember, if what you are doing is working, stick to it. If you stall, make a small change and monitor for ten days to determine if the change had a positive impact on your goals.

This is a common question because fat is so satisfying and often you feel too full to eat any more. This is a great problem to have, in my opinion, because so many diets have the opposite effect.

Missing your target macro goal (by going over or under) for one day is no big deal. However, consistently going over or under can cause issues down the road. A common mistake I see with beginners is that they think if they eat less they will lose more, so they take advantage of the full feeling they are experiencing from the increase in fats and skip meals. While this sounds like a great idea, it can actually result in slowing your metabolism and cause a plateau.

> *A common mistake I see with beginners is that they think if they eat less they will lose more.*

Your goal should always be to come as close as possible to your daily macro goals while granting yourself grace on the days you are a little above or below.

What If I Am Still Hungry?

While this is a less common issue, it is still something I have seen in my experience. If you have eaten all of your food for the day and are still hungry, I would first suggest you discern whether it is real hunger or "head" hunger. One trick I use is to ask myself, "Am I hungry enough to eat plain chicken breast?" If the answer is yes, then start with making a small snack (even if you go above your macro limit). If the answer is no, you may just be battling cravings.

Another way to prevent hunger and stay within your macro goals is to look at how dense your food is. Adding a salad with a small amount of dressing is a great filler that can make you feel more full.

Discern whether it is real hunger or "head" hunger.

Depending on your body's daily caloric expenditure, you may need to make a slight increase in your daily macros. If you are consistently finding you are hungry, listen to your body. Start by increasing your fat macro by 10 percent for a ten-day period and monitor your energy levels, hunger levels, and weight. If the scale is still going down and you are feeling satisfied, then allow this to be a permanent change.

How Often Should I Weigh In?

Some days the number on the scale goes up, and some days the number goes down. On both of those days you are making progress.

The best answer is to weigh in once a week, because the day-to-day fluctuations reported by the scale can be defeating and derail your overall progress. However, I would be lying to you if I told you I have ever consistently weighed in once per week.

What truly needs to happen is that we need to change the meaning we give to the number on the scale. Some days the number on the scale goes up, and some days the number goes down. On both of those days you are making progress. But if you are a daily weigher, I would

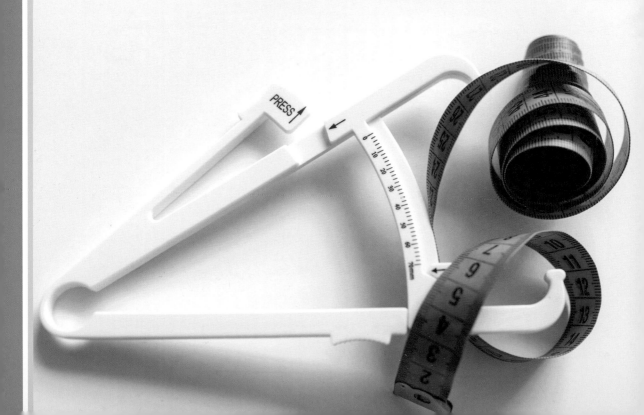

encourage you to use an upward fluctuation in weight to identify foods that possibly are triggering an inflammatory or water-retention reaction.

Our bodies can carry up to nine pounds of water at any given time. *Nine pounds!* So a slight gain could simply be caused by the normal fluctuations in a woman's menstrual cycle. However, you can also look at your food log from the prior day and try to identify foods that caused stalls.

AVOIDING TRIGGERS

Here are some of the biggest trigger-food culprits for fluctuations:

- Sugar replacements
- Dairy
- Alcohol
- Gluten
- Hydrogenated oils
- Vegetable oils
- Processed meats

If you start to see a trend between a certain food and a daily spike on the scale, don't fret. Try eliminating that food for a little while to see how it impacts your overall progress.

· · · · · · · · · ·

Whew! That was a lot of powerful information to take in. If you are feeling a little overwhelmed, it's okay. That's totally normal. Remember, this is a marathon, not a sprint. You can—and you will—begin to build these new habits and discover the hero that's been waiting inside you all along.

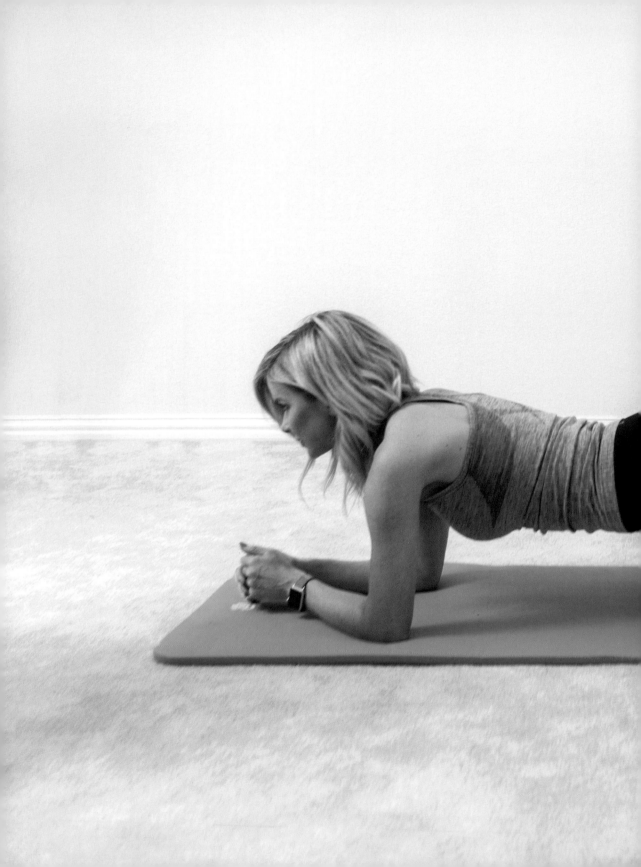

PART 3

THE HEART OF
THE WORKOUT

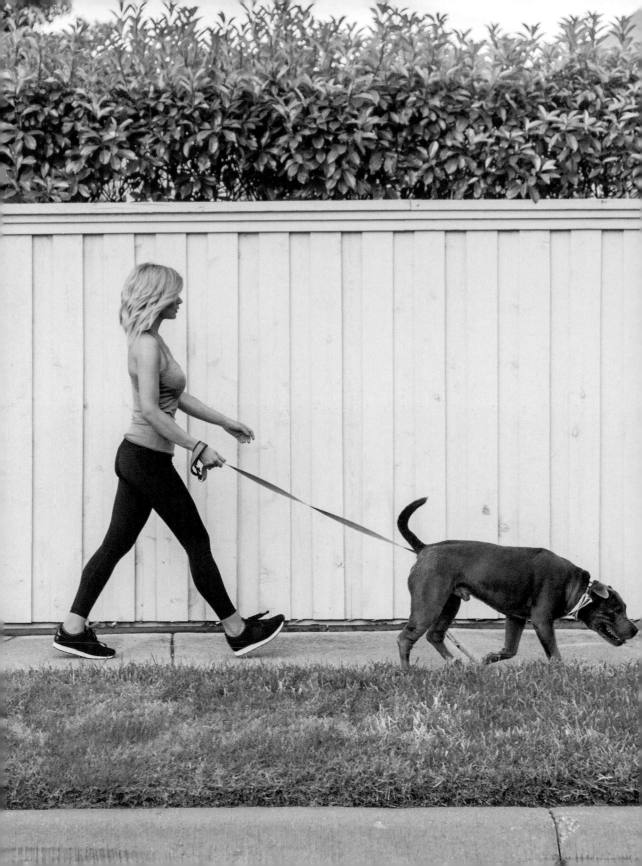

9

GETTING INTO ACTION

When I began my journey, I had a dream I would turn into a cool Zumba teacher, a yoga instructor, and a fitness enthusiast who had a passion for exercise. I always thought I would become a gym freak who spent countless hours perfecting her body each day.

I have a confession to make: I. Hate. Working. Out.

There, I said it. I hate working out! (Whew, that felt good to get off my chest.) And you know what? That's okay! Even though I don't enjoy exercise, I do enjoy the benefits I gain from the process. Just like I don't enjoy brushing my teeth, I understand that if I want pearly whites, I've gotta take care of them.

You don't have to become a couch-potato-turned-fitness-freak overnight. You simply have to decide that it's a small (yet important) piece of a larger process to creating the best version of you!

Why Exercise Matters

It's no secret that exercise is an important part of any weight-loss regimen, but I want to dive deeper into exactly why working out is so important.

If you are like me, you understand how it feels to find yourself repeatedly falling into the mind-set of, "Maybe I should lose the weight first and *then* exercise." Hindsight being twenty-twenty, I realize that thought process makes so much sense because we have always been led to believe that muscle weighs more than fat. And that statement is partially true. While one pound of muscle and one pound of fat are both . . . one pound, because muscle is so dense, it takes up *far* less room on our body than one pound of fat.

My real fear was that if I started exercising the scale might not go down as quickly as I hoped and I would feel discouraged. But remember, this is *not* about a number on the scale. If you were to begin an intense weight-lifting regimen, you would only be adding about half a pound a week! (And that is if you were going all out.) This process of losing weight is about getting our life back, feeling confident, and being *free*.

By adding muscle to our body, we are literally turning ourselves into a fat-burning machine.

I want to start with what science tells us about working out and how it impacts us from a physical perspective.

Whether you are weightlifting or taking a cardio class, exercise has many important benefits, including:

- Weight loss
- Improvement of health conditions
- Reduced depression
- Increased energy
- Better sleep

More than just the overall health benefits, regular exercise turbo-charges your metabolism to help you burn fat more effectively. The more lean muscle we carry on our body, the more effectively we burn calories—even when we're sleeping. By adding muscle to our body, we are literally turning ourselves into a fat-burning machine.

THIS JOURNEY IS SO MUCH MORE THAN REACHING A GOAL WEIGHT.

Working Out and Weight Gain

The common misconception is that adding muscle will make you gain weight. From a technical perspective, that can be true. You technically are gaining weight in the form of muscle. But remember, the goal is to gain a small amount of muscle while simultaneously losing a moderate amount of body fat.

Our mentality about the scale is completely wrong. We have become so focused on a number on the scale that we place its importance over everything. If the scale goes up, we decide the process isn't worth it. If the scale goes down, it must be working!

But how important is the scale really? Do you walk around with your current weight written on your sleeve? Do you update your Facebook status with your current weight each morning? No. Of course not.

We have to change the script in our heads and discover that this journey is so much more than reaching a goal weight. Continue to remind yourself it's about a goal *life*. And that life starts with what we do each and every day.

How to Start a Workout Program

First things first, there is no perfect exercise plan that works for everyone. It simply doesn't exist. Part of this process is finding a style of exercise that you can consistently perform to get your body moving.

I think everyone needs a combination of resistance training and cardio. So often, women automatically focus only on cardio. The problem is no one is going to develop long and lean muscle with cardio alone.

SOME GREAT OPTIONS TO HELP BUILD AND SCULPT LEAN MUSCLES ARE:

- Yoga
- Pilates
- Boot camps
- Dance classes
- Circuit training
- Weightlifting
- Sports like tennis or basketball

The best part about working out is you can try all kinds of different approaches until you find the one you enjoy. I have found that websites like Groupon are fantastic places to find a discounted trial-pass so you can experiment with a new workout method. Many fitness facilities also offer free visits so you can try out a gym and see if it fits you.

Learning to love yourself is one of the most difficult journeys you can embark on, and also one of the most rewarding. You may not see it now, but choosing to improve your health and well-being is a huge factor in developing the self-love you are working on cultivating.

Each time you make an appointment with yourself to work out, to nurture and strengthen your body—and you show up—you are choosing self-love. That's why this process of working out is so critical. It's not just about the physical side—it's about joining the physical, spiritual, and emotional components of your life all together.

Starting Small

When I first started working out, I weighed 297 pounds. There were a lot of workouts I simply could not do because of the amount of weight I was carrying. My knees hurt. My back ached. The thought of getting off my couch and moving my body was more overwhelming than I can say. But you have to start somewhere, and it's okay to start small.

To start out, I dedicated myself to a ten-minute walk each day—no excuses. It's ten minutes! Everyone has ten minutes and a pair of shoes. I promised myself that no matter how tired I was, I was going to prioritize my health and go on that walk.

My daily ten-minute walk turned into fifteen minutes, which turned into thirty minutes. As I began to lose weight, I began to gain the energy I needed to do even more. I found I was less tired and my knees didn't ache as much.

Before long, I finally felt brave enough to take a Zumba class. When I started, I could last for only ten minutes. I was embarrassed to leave the class early, and I always wondered what other people thought of me. But eventually, I realized the only thing that truly mattered was what I thought about myself. I was showing up. I wasn't giving up. I was determined to be better.

MOVE

YOUR

BODY.

> *The key to getting started is simple: get started.*

The key to getting started is simple: *get started*. Move your body. For you, it may be choosing to take the stairs instead of the elevator. You could park farther from the entrance to the store. You could walk a lap around your office building on a break.

Please hear me when I say it doesn't matter how bad you think you are when you start. The whole point is to get started moving your body and to implement this as a daily habit in your routine. You must decide that exercise is a nonnegotiable. You won't get where you want to be unless you do the things required to get there.

Overcoming Fear

My first day at the gym didn't go well. In fact, it didn't go . . . at all.

I was looking for a personal trainer and had been referred to a small, local gym. I had so many fears. My head told me things like, *What if everyone stares at me? What if I'm the biggest person there? What if I don't do it right? Will everyone think I'm stupid?*

Despite all of these thoughts rushing through my mind, I decided to put my fears to rest and go anyway. I got dressed in my typical workout disguise: all-black, loose-fitting clothes. My goal was to look and feel as invisible as possible. I grabbed my water bottle and got in the car.

When I pulled up, I was shocked. When I say this gym was small, I need you to understand—*this gym was small*. There would be no hiding here. I would be exposed for all the fitness fanatics to see.

As I looked inside the glass walls of this gym, I saw two trainers standing at the front in the most intimidating fashion. Their bodies were perfect. Their clothes accentuated every muscle they had spent so long crafting. I didn't know much, but I knew one thing: they will never understand me. I mean, there was no way these people could get it, right? I hated the skin I was in so much, and I wanted to change it. But I was convinced these people with their perfect bodies wouldn't understand where I was.

Despite all of these thoughts rushing through my mind, I decided to put my fears to rest and go anyway.

So, what did I do? I froze. For about thirty minutes I stared blankly at all of the perfect physiques working out and looked down at myself, disgusted with what I saw.

And then . . . I left. Ashamed. Defeated.

As the days passed, I could not shake the feeling inside of me that I simply couldn't give up. I promised myself—not this time. I reached out to the trainer, scheduled an appointment, and learned something new: this was exactly where I belonged.

I realized that for years I had been telling myself a lie: "I didn't belong in the gym. The gym is only for fit people." That. Is. A. Lie. The gym is for people like you and me who simply want to be better, stronger, and healthier. It doesn't matter how you look or what you weigh. What matters is that you have a dream life you are chasing after every single day.

If you are afraid to go to a gym, you aren't alone. It can feel so overwhelming and frightening at first. But here's a word on the fitness gurus you'll meet: they all started somewhere. Maybe they never struggled with weight, but almost all those with great physiques have a story of why they started and why they didn't give up.

How to Enjoy Working Out

As a self-confessed workout hater, I get it. Working out is hard. It's sweaty. It's messy. And it's not nearly as enjoyable as curling up on the couch with your dog and watching your favorite TV show.

Since I hate the actual act of working out, I had to develop techniques to make the process feel a little more bearable.

I started with my actual image.

I started with my actual image. There is so much power and truth behind the saying, "Dress for the job you want." Its fundamental meaning is to dress the part. During my journey, I transitioned from wearing the crappiest clothes I had to actually making gym clothes an important part of my wardrobe. I went out and bought a couple of outfits that made me feel good. I grabbed some new athletic shoes. For you, it might be a fancy fitness watch. Anything you can do to make yourself feel a little more fab during a challenging process is a step in the right direction.

I also became committed to making friends and connections at the gym. I slowly got to know the people around me, and some of those people became my biggest supporters during a difficult time. Before I knew it, going to the gym included feeling cute and seeing friends, which is so much more tolerable than going just to get sweaty and messy.

DRESS
FOR THE
JOB YOU
WANT.

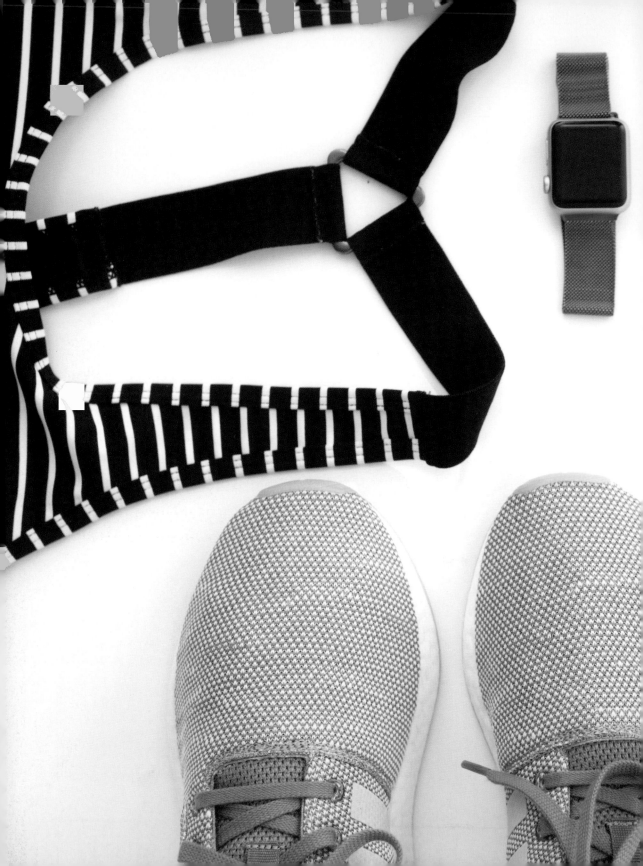

10

WORKOUT 101

Just the idea of working out can feel so overwhelming. With a plethora of information available at our fingertips, it's difficult to know where to even begin.

In the pages that follow, you will find a twenty-eight-day workout plan. This plan is particularly geared for those who are brand-new to working out—or haven't worked out in a while—and are looking for some guidance on how to healthily reestablish a regimen.

You can do a quick Internet search to learn how to properly perform the movements in each of the exercises listed in the four-week workout plan. The only equipment you'll need are three- to five-pound weights and your body.

Now, all you need to do is get started—right where you are, and just as you are. Are you ready?

GETTING STARTED

Here are a few tips to keep in mind as you begin:

1. *Start slow.* So often we hear, "No pain, no gain." This mantra leads us to believe we must endlessly torture ourselves in order to see results. I believe the opposite to be true. Easing into a workout routine gives your body time to adapt and adjust and makes you much more likely to stick to it.

2. *Listen to your body.* If a movement or circuit becomes too difficult, take a break. You can always increase your intensity on the following day. There is no point in exercising to the point of injury because it will result in weeks of not exercising at all.

3. *Breathe.* Make sure you always engage the core muscles of the abdomen and back, and be sure to breathe continuously throughout the workout. Deep breaths ensure oxygen flow and help prevent injury.

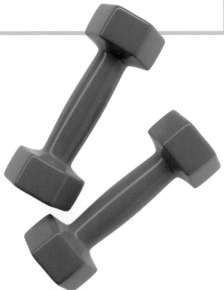

There are two different phases of workouts intended for those who are newer to exercise to help begin building strength and cardiovascular endurance. In these phases, we are performing movements in a *circuit*, which means we are performing one movement after another, without rest, continuously, for the time designated. By doing the movements back-to-back without rest, we are also adding a cardio element along with resistance training.

Remember, even though these sequences are written with no rest periods, you should always rest if you feel the movements are too difficult. After getting the hang of completing the individual circuits, your next goal will be to work your way up to the four-week workout schedule detailed in the pages to come.

For the workouts, going slow and controlled is key to preventing injury. Each repetition should take four to five seconds total to complete. Be sure you are not holding your breath and continue to breathe throughout the movements.

If you are just beginning to work out, I would suggest starting with three-pound dumbbells. If you feel that these workouts are not challenging enough, you can slowly increase the amount of weight used. After the completion of this workout plan, you can continue repeating weeks three and four, and then add an additional challenge by slowly increasing the amount of weight used.

Now, let's get to sweatin'!

Going slow and controlled is key to preventing injury.

WEEK ONE

Starting with the first movement, perform the designated number of reps listed and immediately move to the next movement. There should be no rest taken (unless needed) until the entire time limit for the circuit has been completed. Cardio should be performed immediately following the completion of the circuit.

DAY ONE

Repeat entire circuit for 5 minutes.

20 reps each:

- Squats
- Bicep curls
- Side raises

Cardio: 5 minutes walking at a moderate pace

DAY TWO

Cardio: 10 minutes walking at a moderate pace

DAY THREE

Repeat entire circuit for 5 minutes.

20 reps each:

- Squats
- Bicep curls
- Side raises

Cardio: 5 minutes walking at a moderate pace

DAY FOUR

Cardio: 10 minutes walking at a moderate pace

DAY FIVE

Repeat entire circuit for 5 minutes.

20 reps each:

- Squats
- Bicep curls
- Side raises

Cardio: 5 minutes walking at a moderate pace

WEEK TWO

Starting with the first movement, perform the designated number of reps listed and immediately move to the next movement. There should be no rest taken (unless needed) until the entire time limit for the circuit has been completed.

DAY ONE

Repeat entire circuit for 10 minutes.

20 reps each:

- Squats
- Bicep curls
- Side raises
- 30 seconds rest
- Wall sits (20 seconds each)
- Calf raises
- Bent-over dumbbell rows

DAY TWO

Cardio: 15 minutes walking at a moderate pace

DAY THREE

Repeat entire circuit for 10 minutes.

20 reps each:

- Squats
- Bicep curls
- Side raises
- 30 seconds rest
- Wall sits (20 seconds each)
- Calf raises
- Bent-over dumbbell rows

DAY FOUR

Cardio: 15 minutes walking at a moderate pace

DAY FIVE

Repeat entire circuit for 10 minutes.

20 reps each:

- Squats
- Bicep curls
- Side raises
- 30 seconds rest
- Wall sits (20 seconds each)
- Calf raises
- Bent-over dumbbell rows

WEEK THREE

Starting with the first movement, perform the designated number of reps listed and immediately move to the next movement. There should be no rest taken (unless needed) until the entire time limit for the circuit has been completed.

DAY ONE

Repeat entire circuit for 15 minutes.
20 reps each:

- Squats
- Bicep curls
- Side raises
- Wall sits (20 seconds each)
- 30 seconds rest
- Calf raises
- Bent-over dumbbell rows
- Tricep kickbacks
- Shoulder presses
- Lunges (10 reps per leg)

DAY TWO

Cardio: 20 minutes walking at a moderate pace

DAY THREE

Repeat entire circuit for 15 minutes.
20 reps each:

- Squats
- Bicep curls
- Side raises
- Wall sits (20 seconds each)
- 30 seconds rest
- Calf raises
- Bent-over dumbbell rows
- Tricep kickbacks
- Shoulder presses
- Lunges (10 reps per leg)

DAY FOUR

Cardio: 20 minutes walking at a moderate pace

DAY FIVE

Repeat entire circuit for 15 minutes.
20 reps each:

- Squats
- Bicep curls
- Side raises
- Wall sits (20 seconds each)
- 30 seconds rest
- Calf raises
- Bent-over dumbbell rows
- Tricep kickbacks
- Shoulder presses
- Lunges (10 reps per leg)

WEEK FOUR

Starting with the first movement, perform the designated number of reps listed and immediately move to the next movement. There should be no rest taken (unless needed) until the entire time limit for the circuit has been completed.

DAY ONE

Repeat entire circuit for 20 minutes.
20 reps each:

- Squats
- Bicep curls
- Side raises
- Wall sits (20 seconds each)
- 30 seconds rest

- Calf raises
- Bent-over dumbbell rows
- Tricep kickbacks
- Shoulder presses
- 30 seconds rest

- Lunges (10 reps per leg)
- Wall push-ups
- Front raises
- Fire hydrants (10 reps per leg)

DAY TWO

Cardio: 25 minutes walking at a moderate pace

DAY THREE

Repeat entire circuit for 20 minutes.
20 reps each:

- Squats
- Bicep curls
- Side raises
- Wall sits (20 seconds each)
- 30 seconds rest

- Calf raises
- Bent-over dumbbell rows
- Tricep kickbacks
- Shoulder presses
- 30 seconds rest

- Lunges (10 reps per leg)
- Wall push-ups
- Front raises
- Fire hydrants (10 reps per leg)

DAY FOUR

Cardio: 25 minutes walking at a moderate pace

DAY FIVE

Repeat entire circuit for 20 minutes.
20 reps each:

- Squats
- Bicep curls
- Side raises
- Wall sits (20 seconds each)
- 30 seconds rest

- Calf raises
- Bent-over dumbbell rows
- Tricep kickbacks
- Shoulder presses
- 30 seconds rest

- Lunges (10 reps per leg)
- Wall push-ups
- Front raises
- Fire hydrants (10 reps per leg)

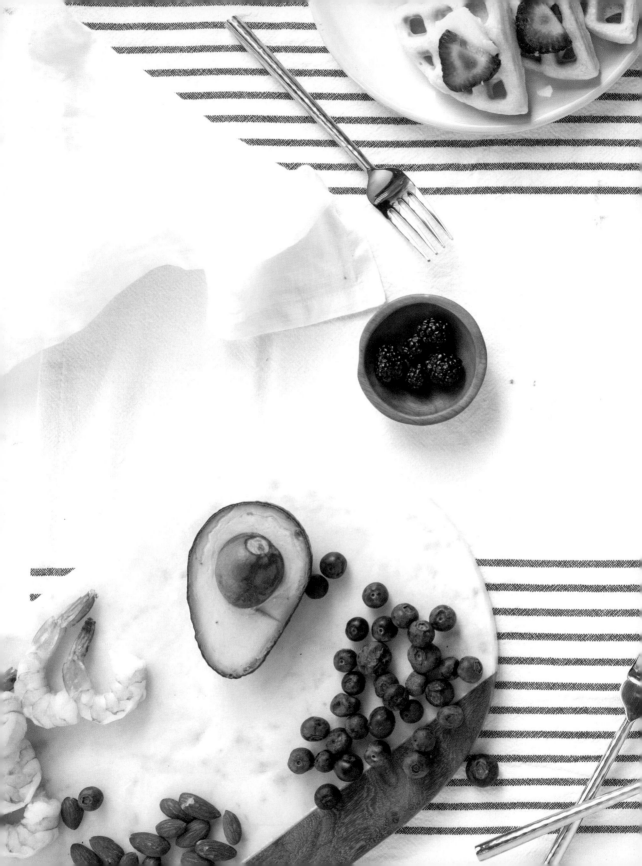

PART 4

SHOPPING LISTS, MEAL PLANS, AND RECIPES

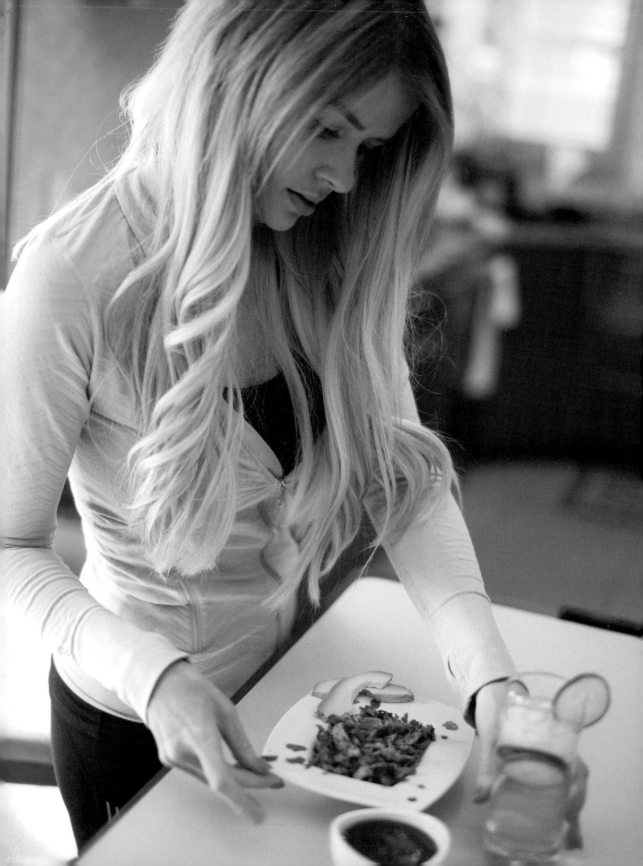

11

FUELING YOUR BODY

Now that we have gained an understanding of how to strengthen
your body, it's time to learn how to fuel it, and begin to understand
exactly *what* you should eat. The shopping list, meal plans, recipes, and
restaurant-ordering guidelines you'll find in this section are designed to
give you an overall picture of the kinds of foods to fill your plate with.

The overall goal of this plan is simplicity. We live in a world centered
around convenience, and I think that's one of the key reasons a lot of diet
plans fail us. When we are required to spend hours a day in the kitchen
cooking complicated meals, our tendency is to give up, ditch our cooking
plans, and head straight to the drive-through. Even if that *is* what happens,
the restaurant section provided in Chapter 14 will help guide you on the
best choices to make.

The other key to this section is finding foods you actually enjoy. For so
many years, I would follow diets full of foods I didn't like. Sure, I could stick to

The overall goal of this plan is simplicity.

a diet for a week or so, but it was only a matter of time before my cravings would become a giant I couldn't slay.

One tip I found to be helpful is to pick four or five favorite recipes you want to nail down. When you feel the urge to fall back on old habits, promise yourself that you'll eat one of your favorite satisfying meals first. Usually, once we eat foods we really enjoy and our hunger is curbed, we are in a much stronger position to stay on track.

I'm so ready for you to begin, I can't wait! I encourage you to go through the entire section and make notes of the recipes and restaurant choices you want to try. Your new beginning starts here, in part four!

Grocery Shopping

This grocery shopping list doesn't include every item you might enjoy, but it is a general overview of foods to look for. If it's on the list, it's good to go. If it's not on the list, be sure to check the food label and make certain it fits the diet goals for the phase you are in.

Protein

Bacon	Pork: pork chops,	Seafood: tuna,	crab, lobster, or
Bone broth	pork tenderloin,	salmon,	oysters
Chicken	or pork ribs	flounder,	Sliced deli meat
Ground beef	Protein shake	snapper, trout,	Steak
Ham	Roast/stew meat	bass, catfish,	Turkey
Lamb, veal, or bison	Sausage	shrimp, scallops,	Whole eggs

Veggies

Artichokes	Celery	Eggplant	Scallions and
Asparagus	Cilantro	Garlic	chives
Avocado	Cucumbers	Green beans	Spaghetti squash
Bell peppers	Dark leafy greens:	Lettuce (all kinds)	Summer squash
Broccoli	spinach, chard,	Mushrooms	Tomato
Brussels sprouts	kale, mustard	Onions	Zucchini
Cabbage	greens, collard	Radishes	
Cauliflower	greens	Sauerkraut	

Fats and Oils

Avocado oil	Cocoa butter	Ghee	Olive oil
Butter	Coconut oil	Lard/tallow	Walnut oil

Dairy

Cheese: Cheddar,	whole-milk	halloumi, and	Sour cream
Swiss, blue,	mozzarella,	full-fat cream	Whipped cream
Gouda, Colby,	mascarpone,	cheese	
provolone,	brie, Gruyere,	Heavy whipping	
feta, parmesan,	goat cheese,	cream	

Nuts and Seeds

Almonds	Chia seeds	Pecans	Pine nuts
Brazil nuts	Hemp heart seeds	Pili nuts	Sunflower seeds
Cashews	Macadamia nuts	Pistachios	Walnuts

Nut Butters

Almond butter	Peanut butter	butter
Cashew butter	Macadamia nut	Sunflower butter

Dairy-Free

Almond milk	whipped cream	Coconut milk	Ripple
Almond or	Califia Farms	Coconut cream	Soy milk
coconut	Cashew milk	Milkadamia	

159

Seasonings

Basil

Chili powder

Cinnamon

Curry

Flavor God
  Seasoning

Garlic powder

Garlic salt

Ginger

Onion powder

Oregano

Paprika

Thyme

Turmeric

Beverages

Bone broth,
  chicken or beef

Carbonated water

(unsweetened)

Coffee, black

Crystal Light

Tea
  (unsweetened),
  black, green, or

herbal

Water

Zevia soda

Condiments/Dressings

Note: All dressings and condiments should have <2 grams of carbs per serving.

Bragg's Liquid
  Aminos

Coconut aminos
  (soy-free and
  gluten-free)

Dressings (full fat):
  ranch, Caesar,

blue cheese,
  or southwest
  chipotle

Fish sauce

Guacamole

Ketchup, reduced
  sugar

Mayonnaise

Mustard (regular
  or spicy)

Pesto

Pickle relish

Marinara sauce

Sugar-free BBQ

sauce

Red wine vinegar

Soy sauce

Sriracha

Sugar-free syrup

Extras

Apple cider
  vinegar

Bragg's Nutritional
  Yeast

Carob powder

Cocoa powder,
  unsweetened

Coconut or
  almond flour

Extracts

Halo Top ice
  cream

Lily's Stevia
  Sweetened

Chocolate

Miracle Noodles

Mission Carb
  Balance soft
  tortilla, 4g net
  carbs

Sugar-free coffee

syrups

Sugar-free
  pudding

Sugar-free gum

Unsweetened
  shredded
  coconut

Natural Sweeteners

Allulose

Erythritol

Monk fruit (liquid
  or powder)

Stevia Glycerite
  liquid

Snacks

Beef jerky	Jimmy Dean	Pork rinds	Tuna, chicken, or
Cheese sticks	Scrambles	Precooked bacon	egg salad
Cheese Whisps	Nuts	Premade salad	
Dill pickles	Olives	Prosciutto	
Hard-boiled eggs	Pepperoni slices	Sliced veggies	

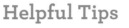

Helpful Tips

Whenever possible, purchase high-quality, organic, cage free meats and dairy, including grass-fed beef and butter, and uncured nitrate-free bacon and sausage (such as Polish or kielbasa). For variety, try hamburger patties such as jalapeño, cheddar, or cowboy.

For an easy meal, buy a rotisserie chicken. And look for fattier cuts for both chicken and for steak, such as T-bone, ribeye, or New York cut. Be sure to check the carb count when shopping for any items, and pay close attention with items such as protein powder, ham, or flavored almonds.

For extra fat, add add butter or heavy whipping cream to bone broth or coffee, or use coconut oil for cooking.

Try using Mission Carb Balance soft tortillas to make wraps, tacos, or pizza.

Some of my other favorite brands include:

Mayonnaise: Primal Kitchen

Marinara Sauce: Rao's

Guacamole: Wholly Guacamole

Soy Sauce: Tamari (gluten-free)

Sugar-free syrup: Walden Farms or Lakanto

Erythritol: Swerve

Stevia glycerite liquid: Sweet Drops

161

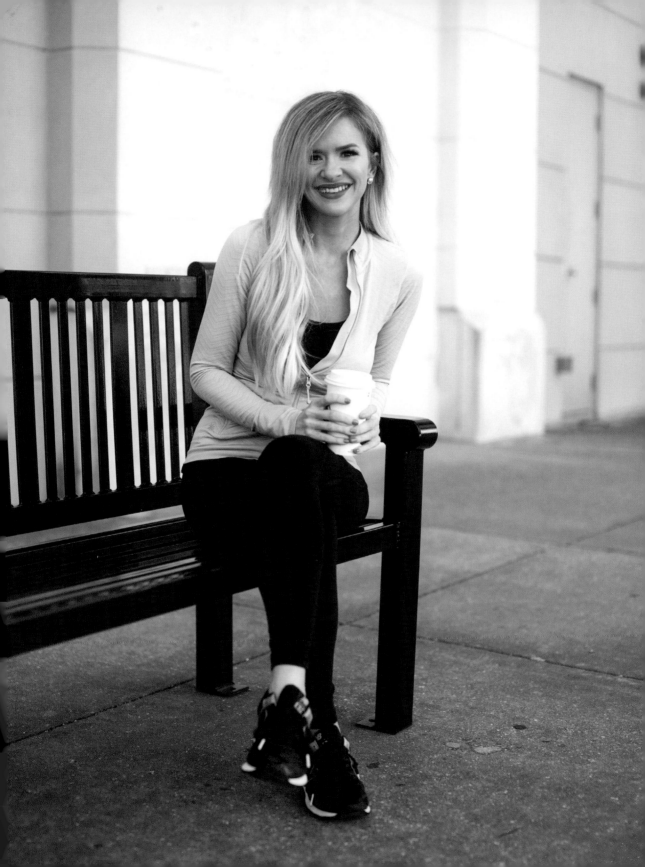

12

MEAL PLANS

One thing you will notice in the meal plan examples that I'm providing is a heavy amount of repetition. This is by design. You may not realize it, but even now you probably eat a lot of the same foods on repeat.

I saw my greatest success when I generally rotated a lot of the same meals, then occasionally tried something new to shake things up a bit. You can find all of the recipes in the next chapter.

On the following pages, I've provided a Standard Keto One-Month Meal Plan to get you started. This can be used with diet phases one and two, found in Chapter 6. To add extra fat to any of the low-fat dishes, try adding a little mayonnaise, half of an avocado, or sour cream. Remember to keep a log of the food and how it makes you feel, and then adjust as necessary.

WEEK ONE

SUNDAY

Breakfast: Scrambled Eggs and Avocado

Lunch: Tuna Salad

Can be served in lettuce cups or low-carb tortillas.

Dinner: Salsa Chicken

Can be served in lettuce cups or low-carb tortillas.

MONDAY

Breakfast: Eggs and Bacon

Lunch: Tuna Salad

Can be served in lettuce cups or low-carb tortillas.

Dinner: Salsa Chicken

Can be served in lettuce cups or low-carb tortillas.

TUESDAY

Breakfast: Sausage, Egg, and Cheese Melt

Lunch: Salad Bowl

Dinner: Pork Rind Nachos

WEDNESDAY

Breakfast: Scrambled Eggs and Avocado

Lunch: Egg Salad

> *Can be served in lettuce cups or low-carb tortillas.*

Dinner: Taco Bowl

THURSDAY

Breakfast: Eggs and Bacon

Lunch: Egg Salad

> *Can be served in lettuce cups or low-carb tortillas.*

Dinner: Low-Carb Pizza

FRIDAY

Breakfast: Eggs, Sausage, and Cheese Melt

Lunch: Big Mac Salad

Dinner: Shrimp Fried Cauliflower Rice

SATURDAY

Breakfast: Scrambled Eggs and Avocado

Lunch: Shrimp Fried Cauliflower Rice

Dinner: Burger Bowl

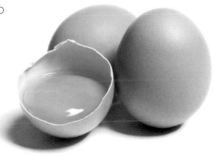

———— WEEK TWO ————

SUNDAY

Breakfast: Vanilla Overnight "Oats"

Lunch: Ham and Cheese Roll-ups

Dinner: Cheesy BBQ Bacon Meatballs and Cauliflower Mac-n-Cheese

MONDAY

Breakfast: Protein shake with 1 tablespoon melted coconut oil

Lunch: Salad Bowl

Dinner: Shrimp Fried Cauliflower Rice

TUESDAY

Breakfast: 90-Second Bread with a side of bacon

Lunch: Beef and Broccoli Stir-Fry

Dinner: Inside-Out Egg Roll

WEDNESDAY

Breakfast: Breakfast Bowl

Lunch: Inside-Out Egg Roll

Dinner: Beef and Broccoli Stir-Fry

THURSDAY

Breakfast: Breakfast Sausage Balls

Lunch: Grilled chicken and Creamed Spinach

Dinner: Cheesy BBQ Bacon Meatballs and Cauliflower Mac-n-Cheese

FRIDAY

Breakfast: Protein shake with 1 tablespoon melted coconut oil

Lunch: Cheesy BBQ Bacon Meatballs and Cauliflower Mac-n-Cheese

Dinner: Volcano Roll in a Bowl

SATURDAY

Breakfast: Breakfast Sausage Balls

Lunch: Quick Cobb Salad

Dinner: Grilled steak and Zesty Broccoli

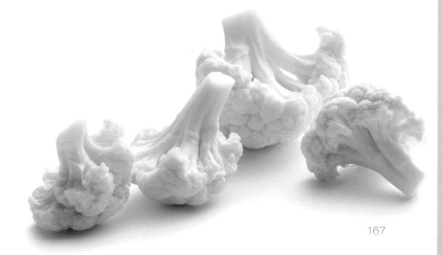

—————— WEEK THREE ——————

SUNDAY

Breakfast: Sausage, Egg, and Cheese Melt

Lunch: Big Mac Salad

Dinner: Low-Carb Pizza

MONDAY

Breakfast: Sausage, Egg, and Cheese Melt

Lunch: Ham and Cheese Roll-ups

Dinner: Inside-Out Egg Roll

TUESDAY

Breakfast: Scrambled Eggs and Avocado

Lunch: Inside-Out Egg Roll

Dinner: BBQ Bacon Meatloaf and Creamed Spinach

WEDNESDAY

Breakfast: Sausage, Egg, and Cheese Melt

Lunch: Inside-Out Egg Roll

Dinner: BBQ Bacon Meatloaf and Creamed Spinach

THURSDAY

Breakfast: Keto Waffles

Lunch: Salsa Chicken

> *Can be served in lettuce cups or low-carb tortillas.*

Dinner: Tuna Salad

> *Can be served in lettuce cups or low-carb tortillas.*

FRIDAY

Breakfast: Eggs and Bacon

Lunch: Tuna Salad

> *Can be served in lettuce cups or low-carb tortillas.*

Dinner: Low-Carb Tacos

SATURDAY

Breakfast: Keto Waffles

Lunch: Salad Bowl

Dinner: Low-Carb Tacos

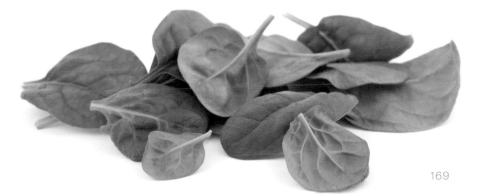

WEEK FOUR

SUNDAY

Breakfast: Scrambled Eggs and Avocado

Lunch: Grilled chicken and Creamed Spinach

Dinner: Burger Bowl

MONDAY

Breakfast: Eggs and Sausage

Lunch: Grilled chicken and Creamed Spinach

Dinner: Volcano Roll in a Bowl

TUESDAY

Breakfast: Sausage, Egg, and Cheese Melt

Lunch: Salad Bowl

Dinner: Taco Soup

WEDNESDAY

Breakfast: Keto Waffles

Lunch: Taco Soup

Dinner: Chicken, Bacon, and Ranch Casserole

THURSDAY

Breakfast: Scrambled Eggs and Avocado

Lunch: Taco Soup

Dinner: Chicken, Bacon, and Ranch Casserole

FRIDAY

Breakfast: Protein shake with 1 tablespoon melted coconut oil

Lunch: Chicken, Bacon, and Ranch Casserole

Dinner: Taco Bowl

SATURDAY

Breakfast: Eggs and Bacon

Lunch: Big Mac Salad

Dinner: Low-Carb Pizza

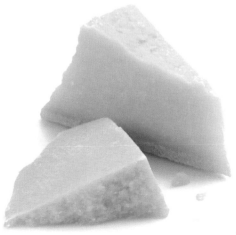

Dairy-Free Keto One-Week Meal Plan

This Meal Plan can be used with Diet Phases 1–4.

SUNDAY

Breakfast: Scrambled Eggs and Avocado

Lunch: Tuna Salad

> *Can be served in lettuce cups or low-carb, gluten-free tortillas.*

Dinner: Salsa Chicken

> *Can be served in lettuce cups or low-carb, gluten-free tortillas.*

MONDAY

Breakfast: Scrambled Eggs and Avocado

Lunch: Tuna Salad

> *Can be served in lettuce cups or low-carb, gluten-free tortillas.*

Dinner: Salsa Chicken

> *Can be served in lettuce cups or low-carb, gluten-free tortillas.*

TUESDAY

Breakfast: Eggs and Sausage

Lunch: Salad Bowl

Dinner: Salsa Chicken

> *Can be served in lettuce cups or low-carb, gluten-free tortillas.*

WEDNESDAY

Breakfast: Scrambled Eggs and Avocado

Lunch: Egg Salad

Can be served in lettuce cups or low-carb, gluten-free tortillas.

Dinner: Taco Bowl

THURSDAY

Breakfast: Eggs and Bacon

Lunch: Egg Salad

Can be served in lettuce cups or low-carb, gluten-free tortillas.

Dinner: Taco Bowl

FRIDAY

Breakfast: Eggs and Sausage

Lunch: Salad Bowl

Dinner: Shrimp Fried Cauliflower Rice

SATURDAY

Breakfast: Scrambled Eggs and Avocado

Lunch: Shrimp Fried Cauliflower Rice

Dinner: Burger Bowl

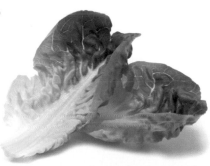

Vegan Keto One-Week Meal Plan

This Meal Plan can be used with Diet Phases 1–4.

SUNDAY

Breakfast: Vegan Breakfast Scramble

Lunch: Vegan Stir-Fry Bowl

Dinner: Cashew Crack Slaw

MONDAY

Breakfast: Vegan Breakfast Scramble

Lunch: Cashew Crack Slaw

Dinner: Vegan Stir-Fry Bowl

TUESDAY

Breakfast: Vegan Breakfast Scramble

Lunch: Cashew Crack Slaw

Dinner: Vegan Salad Bowl

WEDNESDAY

Breakfast: Vanilla Overnight "Oats"

Lunch: Vegan Salad Bowl

Dinner: Mexican Cauliflower Rice

THURSDAY

Breakfast: Vanilla Overnight "Oats"

Lunch: Mexican Cauliflower Rice

Dinner: Vegan Stir-Fry Bowl

FRIDAY

Breakfast: Breakfast Shake

Lunch: Vegan Stir-Fry Bowl

Dinner: Creamy Zucchini Pasta

SATURDAY

Breakfast: Breakfast Shake

Lunch: Creamy Zucchini Pasta

Dinner: Vegan Stir-Fry Bowl

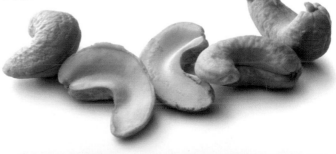

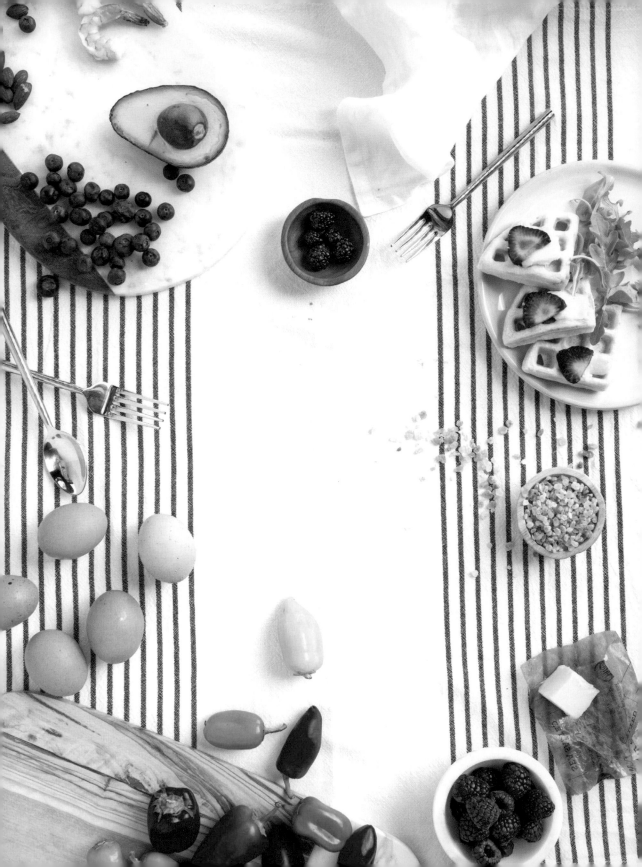

RECIPES

Simple recipes are my jam. When I first started on my road to become healthy, I owned approximately one pan and one spatula—and hadn't the slightest clue how to use them. I have always been the girl who could mess up Easy Mac (thank goodness I don't eat this anymore), and there's something about the term *Easy Mac* that indicates it shouldn't be so challenging.

I felt daunted when I looked at recipes that had what seemed like hundreds of ingredients and required two hours of prep. I had a rule: if there are more than five ingredients, it ain't happening!

Part of this process is embracing the reality that you may not ever be a master chef or a die-hard meal prepper, and that's okay. Instead of trying to force yourself to become something you're not, I have created some of my favorite simple recipes anyone can follow.

Simplicity aside, the other piece of the weight-loss puzzle is finding

Food does not have to be boring and tasteless in order for you to lose weight.

foods you actually enjoy. Understand this: food does not have to be boring and tasteless in order for you to lose weight. It just doesn't. Do you like pizza? Great! I have included an amazing pizza recipe that will satisfy your taste buds while keeping you on track.

I highly suggest picking five or six recipes that you *love* to help you through the rough days when the food cravings just won't quit. When you have an arsenal of meals on hand that satisfy you, that will help you keep from straying from your plan.

In each section, I've also included some of my favorite Build-a-Bowl recipes and they're as simple as they sound. Choose a protein, fat, topping, and dressing from each category. Feel free to mix and match—and explore! The ingredients for each recipe go well with each other. You really can't go wrong.

I'm so excited for you to explore these recipes I have created. I encourage you to try out some of the ones that might not look so appetizing because I think they will surprise you. (Fried green beans probably sound boring, but you have to trust me on this one.)

BREAKFAST

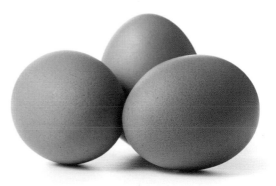

Keto Hot Chocolate

Ingredients

- 3 tablespoons cocoa powder, unsweetened
- 2 tablespoons granular erythritol (Swerve)
- 2 cups almond milk
- 1 cup heavy whipping cream
- $1/4$ teaspoon pure vanilla extract
- Optional: Salt, dash of ground cinnamon, and sugar-free whipped cream

Directions

1. Add cocoa powder, erythritol, almond milk, and heavy whipping cream (and salt if using) to a small saucepan.
2. Heat over medium heat and whisk to combine.
3. Remove from heat and stir in vanilla.
4. Top with cinnamon and sugar-free whipped cream if desired.

Macros per serving: 23g F | 3g P | 3g NC

Makes 4 servings.

Keto Coffee

Ingredients

- 12 ounces organic black coffee
- 1 tablespoon organic coconut oil
- 1 tablespoon grass-fed butter (not margarine)
- $1/2$ teaspoon pure vanilla extract
- 1 to 2 drops liquid stevia

Directions

1. Combine coffee, coconut oil, butter, vanilla, and liquid stevia together in a cup.
2. Mix well with a small whisk and serve.

Macros per serving: 26g F | 0g P | 0g NC

Makes 1 serving.

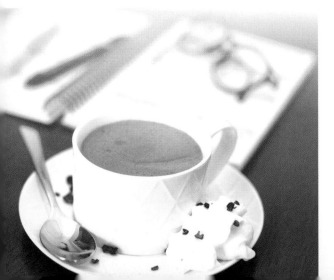

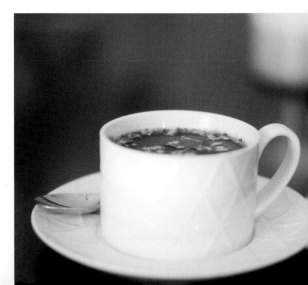

Scrambled Eggs and Avocado

*Dairy-free recipe with modifications

Ingredients

- 2 large eggs
- 1 large egg yolk
- 1 tablespoon butter (or dairy-free vegan butter)
- Salt and black pepper to taste
- Half avocado, sliced

Directions

1. Beat eggs together in a bowl.
2. Melt butter in skillet on medium-high heat.
3. Add eggs, salt, and pepper to pan. Move eggs around until thoroughly cooked. Remove from heat.
4. Top eggs with sliced avocado.

Tip: Adding salt to the avocado adds flavor. Use Icelandic Flake Salt to gain additional electrolytes.

Macros per serving: 36g F | 17g P | 3g NC

Makes 1 serving.

Sausage, Egg, and Cheese Melt

Ingredients

- 8 large eggs
- 2 tablespoons butter (or dairy-free vegan butter)
- 6 ounces sausage
- Salt and black pepper to taste
- $1/2$ cup shredded Cheddar cheese

Directions

1. Beat eggs together in a bowl.
2. Melt butter in skillet on medium-high heat.
3. In a skillet, brown sausage over medium-high heat until thoroughly cooked.
4. In a separate pan, add eggs, salt, and pepper. Move eggs around until thoroughly cooked. Remove from heat.
5. Combine sausage with eggs and top with shredded cheese.

Macros per serving: 44g F | 22g P | 2g NC

Makes 4 servings.

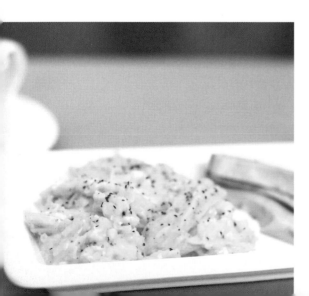

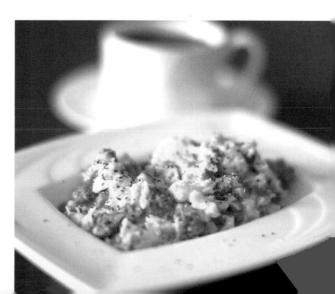

Keto Waffles

Ingredients

3 large eggs

4 ounces whipped cream cheese

1 teaspoon pure vanilla extract

2 tablespoons butter

Sugar-free syrup

Directions

1. Turn on waffle iron to preheat.
2. In a blender or food processor, blend eggs, whipped cream cheese, and vanilla until well combined.
3. Pour into a greased waffle iron until the sections are three-fourths full. Close waffle iron and thoroughly cook. The waffles should be stiff yet soft.
4. Remove from waffle iron and top with butter and sugar-free syrup.

Macros per serving: 22g F | 11g 1P | 5g NC

Makes 2 servings.

Breakfast Sausage Balls

Ingredients

1 large egg

2 teaspoons baking powder

1/2 teaspoon salt

1 pound breakfast sausage

1 cup almond flour

8 ounces shredded Cheddar cheese

1/2 cup grated Parmesan

Directions

1. Preheat oven to 350 degrees.
2. In a small bowl combine egg, baking powder, and salt and whisk together until well combined.
3. In a large bowl add egg mixture, sausage, flour, Cheddar, and Parmesan and combine.
4. Using your hands, make 20 to 25 sausage balls and spread out evenly on cookie sheet.
5. Bake in oven for 16 to 20 minutes until thoroughly cooked.

Macros per serving: 33g F | 18g P | 3g NC

Makes 6 servings.

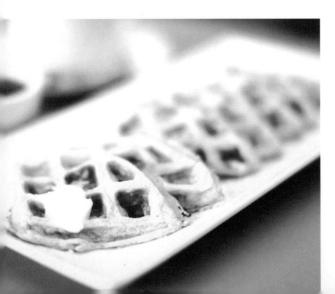

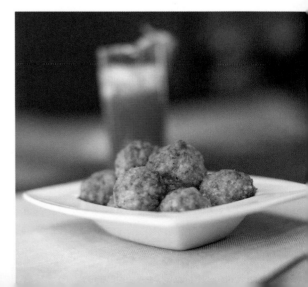

Eggs and Bacon

Ingredients

- 2 large eggs
- 2 strips of bacon
- 1/2 tablespoon butter

Directions

1. This is where you can get creative and prepare the eggs your favorite way: fried, poached, scrambled, over easy, or hard-boiled.
2. Similarly, you can either bake the bacon in an oven or simply pan fry the bacon—and then use the bacon grease to fry your eggs.
3. If baking in an oven, preheat the oven to 400 degrees.
4. Place the strips of bacon on a baking sheet, and bake until the bacon is thoroughly cooked and crispy, about 20 minutes, depending on thickness.

Macros per serving: 22g F | 28g P | 2g NC

Makes 1 serving.

Eggs and Sausage

Ingredients

- 2 large eggs
- 3 ounces of sausage
- 1/2 tablespoon butter

Directions

1. This is where you can get creative and prepare the eggs your favorite way: fried, poached, scrambled, over easy, or hard-boiled.
2. Similarly, choose either ground sausage, sausage links, or patties.
3. Pan fry the sausage—and depending on how you prefer your eggs, you may use the sausage grease to fry your eggs for extra flavor.

Macros per serving: 40g F | 28g P | 2g NC

Makes 1 serving.

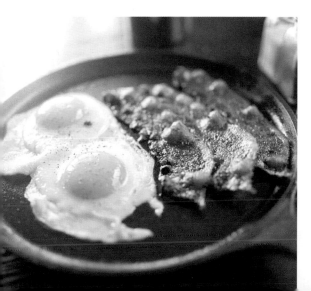

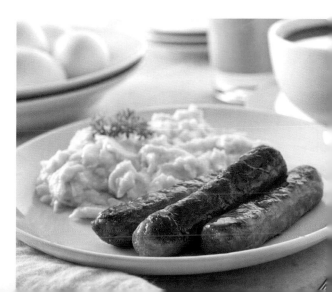

BREAKFAST BOWL

PROTEIN

Food Item	Quantity	Fat	Protein	Net Carbs
Bacon	2 pieces	6g	5g	0g
Sausage	1 ounce	8g	5g	0g
Whole Eggs	2	16g	13g	1g

FATS

Food Item	Quantity	Fat	Protein	Net Carbs
Avocado	1/2	21g	3g	2g
Avocado or Olive Oil	1 tablespoon	14g	0g	0g
Butter	1 tablespoon	12g	0g	0g
Cheddar Cheese	1 ounce	9g	6g	1g
Sour Cream	2 tablespoons	6g	1g	1g

EXTRAS

Food Item	Quantity	Fat	Protein	Net Carbs
Bell Pepper	1/2 cup	0g	1g	2g
Jalapeños	1 tablespoon	0g	0g	0g
Mushrooms	1/4 cup	0g	0g	0g
Onions	2 tablespoons	0g	0g	2g
Salsa	1 tablespoon	0g	0g	1g
Spinach	2 ounces	0g	2g	1g
Low-Carb, Gluten-Free Tortilla	1	2g	3g	3g

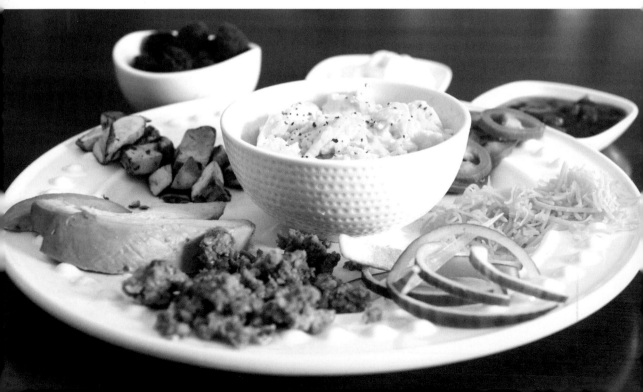

MAIN DISHES

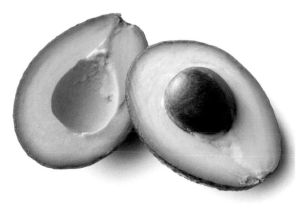

Quick Cobb Salad

Ingredients

- 6 cups romaine lettuce, chopped
- 4 large eggs, hard-boiled, peeled, and chopped
- 1 1/2 cups olives, pitted
- 1 1/2 cups ham deli meat, chopped
- 1/2 cup blue cheese crumbles
- 1 tomato, diced
- 1 small red onion, chopped
- 3/4 cup blue cheese dressing

Directions

1. In a large bowl add lettuce.
2. Add eggs, olives, ham, blue cheese, tomato, and onion, and top with dressing.
3. Mix salad to your liking and enjoy!

Dairy-free option: Sub blue cheese crumbles with dairy-free cheese and sub blue cheese dressing with oil, vinegar, and fresh lemon juice.

Macros per serving: 26g F | 13g P | 7.5g NC

Makes 6 servings.

Big Mac Salad

Ingredients

- 1/2 pound 80/20 ground beef
- 1/4 cup water
- 2 teaspoons Worcestershire sauce
- 1 teaspoon paprika
- 1 teaspoon black pepper
- 1/4 onion, finely diced
- 1 romaine lettuce head, thinly sliced
- 3 baby dill pickles, chopped
- 4 tablespoons shredded Cheddar cheese
- 4 tablespoons Thousand Island dressing
- 2 tablespoons sesame seeds

Directions

1. Over medium heat, cook the ground beef in a pan with the water, Worcestershire, paprika, and pepper until meat is well done.
2. In a separate pan, sauté the onions until translucent.
3. Add beef, onions, lettuce, pickles, cheese, dressing, and sesame seeds to a large bowl and mix.

Macros per serving: 25g F | 25g P | 7g NC

Makes 6 servings.

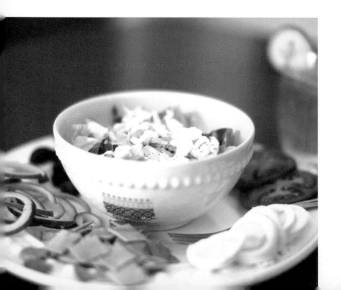

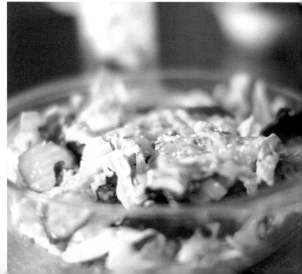

SALAD BOWL

PROTEIN

Food Item	Quantity	Fat	Protein	Net Carbs
Bacon	2 slices	6g	5g	0g
Chicken	3 ounces	4g	26g	0g
Egg	1 whole	8g	6g	1g
Ground Beef	3 ounces	14g	21g	0g
Salmon	3 ounces	11g	19g	0g
Shrimp	3 ounces	0g	20g	0g
Steak	3 ounces	13g	23g	0g

FATS

Avocado	1/2	21g	3g	2g
Almonds	1 ounce	15g	6g	3g
Avocado or Olive Oil	1 tablespoon	14g	0g	0g
Goat Cheese	1 ounce	6g	5g	0g
Shredded Cheese	1 ounce	9g	6g	1g

EXTRAS

Broccoli	1/4 cup	0g	1g	1g
Lettuce	2 cups	0g	0g	2g
Mushrooms	1/4 cup	0g	0g	0g
Onions	2 tablespoons	0g	0g	2g

DRESSINGS

Ranch	2 tablespoons	16g	0g	2g
Caesar	2 tablespoons	17g	0g	1g
Oil and Vinegar	2 tablespoons	16g	0g	1g

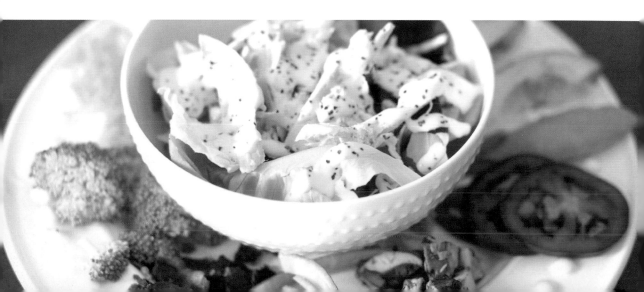

Inside-Out Egg Roll

*Dairy-free recipe

Ingredients

- 1 pound $^{80}/20$ ground beef
- 1 tablespoon sesame oil
- 2 tablespoons olive oil
- $^{1}/2$ cup green onions
- 1 teaspoon minced garlic
- 1 bag shredded cabbage
- 2 tablespoons soy sauce
- 1 teaspoon crushed red pepper

Directions

1. Brown ground beef in pan until thoroughly cooked. Drain excess fat.
2. In a separate pan combine sesame oil, olive oil, green onions, and minced garlic. Fry until tender.
3. Add cabbage and crushed red pepper. Heat until mostly tender.
4. Add in ground beef and onion mixture and combine.

Macros per serving: 28g F | 28g P | 4g NC

Makes 4 servings.

Volcano Roll in a Bowl

*Dairy-free recipe

Ingredients

- 1 tablespoon avocado oil
- 12 precooked shrimp, peeled and deveined
- 4 tablespoons mayonnaise
- 1 tablespoon Sriracha sauce
- 1 cucumber, thinly sliced

Directions

1. In a medium pan heat oil over high heat.
2. Add in shrimp, and cook on each side for 1 to 2 minutes, until warm.
3. Remove pan from heat and stir in mayo and Sriracha with shrimp.
4. Add entire mixture to a bowl and serve with cucumber slices.

Macros per serving: 28g F | 16g P | 3g NC

Makes 4 servings.

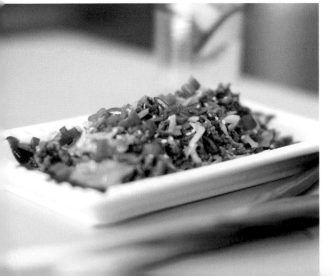 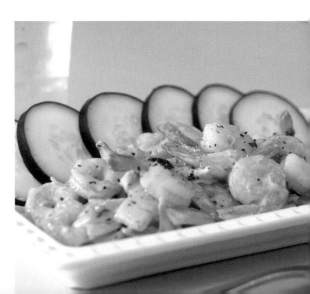

Ham and Cheese Roll-ups

Ingredients

- 3 slices of ham (check carb count)
- 3 slices of Swiss or Cheddar cheese
- 1 tablespoon mayonnaise
- 2 low-carb tortillas

Directions

1. Lay ham and cheese on top of each other to create a layer.
2. Spread thin layer of mayo on top.
3. Roll up the ham and cheese.
4. Slice into bite-size rounds.

Macros per serving: 31g F | 27g P | 2g NC

Makes 1 serving.

Avocado Chicken Salad

*Dairy-free recipe

Ingredients

- 2 (6-ounce) chicken breasts, cooked
- 2 tablespoons avocado or olive oil
- 2 small avocados
- 1/4 cup diced red onion
- 1 tablespoon fresh cilantro
- 1 tablespoon lime juice
- Salt and black pepper to taste

Directions

1. In a medium bowl dice chicken into small, bite-size pieces.
2. In a separate bowl combine oil, avocado, onion, cilantro, lime juice, salt, and pepper. Mash the avocado until smooth.
3. Add avocado mixture to the bowl of diced chicken and combine.

Macros per serving: 20g F | 28g P | 3g NC

Makes 4 servings.

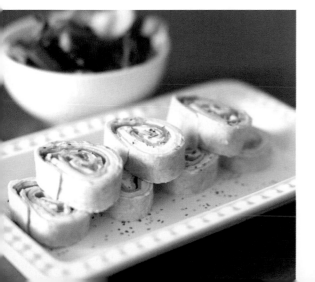

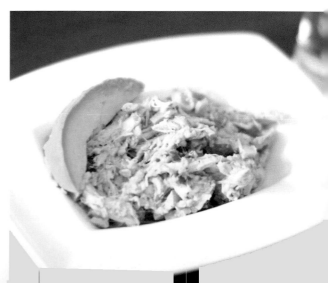

Egg Salad

*Dairy-free recipe

Ingredients

6 large eggs, hard-boiled, chopped

1/4 cup mayonnaise

1/4 cup diced celery

1 tablespoon pickle relish

Salt and black pepper to taste

Garlic powder to taste

Onion powder to taste

Directions

1. Place chopped eggs in a medium-size bowl.
2. Stir in mayo, celery, pickle relish, salt, pepper, garlic powder, and onion powder.
3. This can be eaten by itself or added to lettuce cups or a low-carb tortilla!

Macros per serving: 25g F | 13g P | 2g NC

Makes 3 servings.

Tuna Salad

*Dairy-free recipe

Ingredients

1 can of white tuna in water

2 large eggs, hard-boiled, chopped

3/4 cup mayonnaise

1 tablespoon olive oil

1 teaspoon mustard

1/2 teaspoon garlic salt

1/2 teaspoon onion powder

Salt and black pepper to taste

Directions

1. Drain water from can and place tuna in a bowl.
2. Add in eggs, mayo, olive oil, mustard, garlic salt, onion powder, salt, and pepper, and mix well.
3. This can be eaten by itself or added to lettuce cups or a low-carb tortilla!

Macros per serving: 31g F | 11g P | 1g NC

Makes 5 servings.

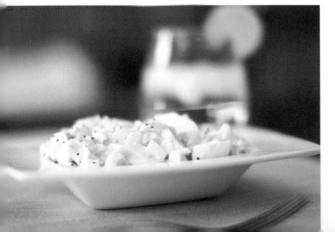

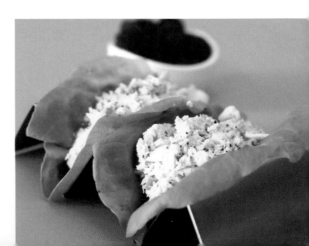

Low-Carb Tacos

*Dairy-free recipe with modifications

Ingredients

1 pound ^{80}/20 ground beef

1 tablespoon chili powder

2 teaspoons cumin

1 teaspoon paprika

1/2 teaspoon garlic powder

1/2 teaspoon onion powder

1/2 teaspoon salt

1/2 teaspoon black pepper

4 large lettuce leaves or low-carb, gluten-free tortillas (under 7g net carbs)

1/4 cup shredded Cheddar cheese (omit if dairy-free)

1/2 avocado, diced

Dash of Sriracha

Directions

1. Heat large skillet over medium-high heat. Add beef and cook until thoroughly cooked. Drain excess liquid.
2. In a small bowl mix together chili powder, cumin, paprika, garlic powder, onion powder, salt, and pepper.
3. Return beef to pan and add taco seasoning mix. Stir.
4. Add hamburger mixture to the tortilla and top with cheese, avocado, and Sriracha.

Macros per serving: 24g F | 31g P | 6g NC

Makes 4 servings.

Taco Soup

Ingredients

2 pounds ^{80}/20 ground beef

1 small onion, diced

2 teaspoons minced garlic

1 can of Ro-Tel Original diced tomatoes and green chilies

1 packet of taco seasoning

1 (8-ounce) package cream cheese

4 cups chicken broth

Shredded Cheddar

Bacon crumbles

Directions

1. Over medium heat, in a skillet, brown ground beef, onion, and minced garlic until thoroughly cooked. Drain excess liquid.
2. In a slow cooker or Instant Pot, combine can diced tomatoes and green chilies, taco seasoning, cream cheese, and chicken broth with the beef mixture.
3. If using a slow cooker, cook on high for 2 hours or on low for 4 hours. If using an Instant Pot, cook at high pressure for 15 minutes.
4. To serve, top with cheese and bacon.

Macros per serving: 17g F | 19g P | 3g NC

Makes 14 servings.

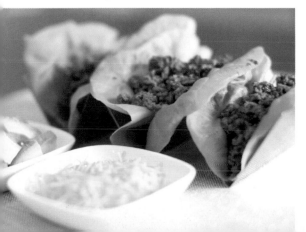
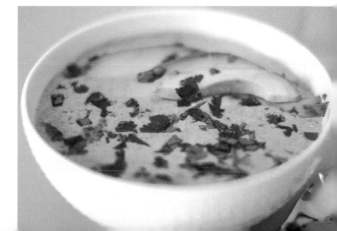

TACO BOWL

PROTEIN

Food Item	Quantity	Fat	Protein	Net Carbs
80/20 Ground Beef	3 ounces	14g	21g	0g
90/10 Ground Beef	3 ounces	9g	23g	0g
Shredded Chicken	3 ounces	4g	26g	0g
Ground Turkey	3 ounces	15g	21g	0g

FATS

Food Item	Quantity	Fat	Protein	Net Carbs
Avocado	1/2	21g	3g	2g
Avocado or Olive Oil	1 tablespoon	14g	0g	0g
Cheddar Cheese	1 ounce	9g	6g	1g
Sour Cream	2 tablespoons	6g	1g	1g

EXTRAS

Food Item	Quantity	Fat	Protein	Net Carbs
Bell Pepper	1/2 cup	0g	1g	2g
Jalapeños	1 tablespoon	0g	0g	0g
Lettuce	1 cup	0g	0g	1g
Mushrooms	1/4 cup	0g	0g	0g
Onions	2 tablespoons	0g	0g	2g
Salsa	1 tablespoon	0g	0g	1g
Low-Carb, Gluten-Free Tortilla	1	2g	3g	3g

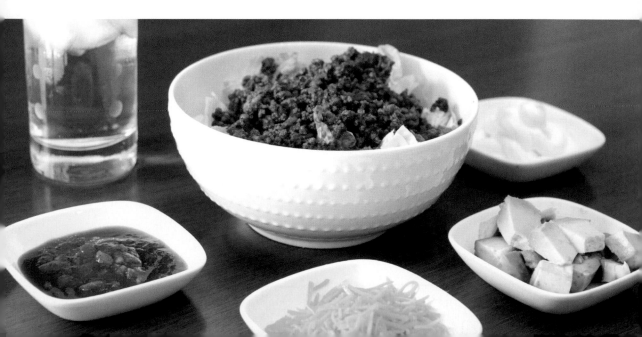

Low-Carb Pizza

Ingredients

- 2 tablespoons marinara or pizza sauce
- 1 low-carb tortilla (under 7g net carbs)
- 1/4 cup shredded mozzarella cheese
- 4 slices pepperoni

Directions

1. Preheat oven to 400 degrees.
2. Spread thin layer of marinara sauce onto the low-carb tortilla.
3. Top with cheese and pepperoni.
4. Bake directly on oven rack for 5 to 6 minutes until cheese is bubbly.

Macros per serving: 23g F | 18g P | 8g NC

Makes 1 serving.

Pork Rind Nachos

Ingredients

- 2 ounces pork rinds
- 1 cup shredded Cheddar cheese
- 10 ounces slow-cooked chicken or beef roast in au jus (I used Hormel brand)
- 1/4 cup black olives, sliced
- 1 tablespoon jalapeños, sliced
- 2 tablespoons salsa
- 2 tablespoons guacamole
- 2 tablespoons sour cream

Directions

1. Set oven to broil.
2. Use foil to cover baking sheet, then spread out pork rinds and top with cheese.
3. Broil until cheese melts, about 3 minutes.
4. Top the rinds and cheese with roast, olives, jalapeños, salsa, guacamole, and sour cream, and enjoy!

Macros per serving: 21.5g F | 29g P | 4g NC

Makes 4 servings.

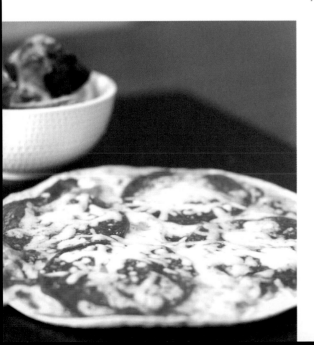

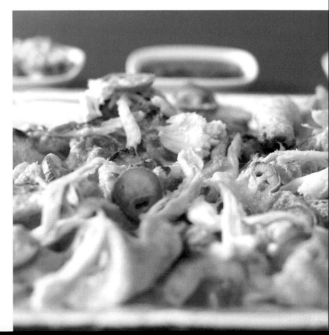

BURGER BOWL

PROTEIN

Food Item	Quantity	Fat	Protein	Net Carbs
Ground Beef	3 ounces	14g	21g	0g
Egg	1 whole	8g	6g	1g
Bacon	2 slices	6g	5g	0g

FATS

Avocado	1/2	21g	3g	2g
Avocado or Olive Oil	1 tablespoon	14g	0g	0g
Goat Cheese	1 ounce	6g	5g	0g
Sliced Cheese	1 ounce	9g	6g	1g

TOPPINGS

Tomato	1/4 cup	0g	0g	1g
Lettuce	2 cups	0g	0g	2g
Mushrooms	1/4 cup	0g	0g	0g
Onions	2 tablespoons	0g	0g	2g

DRESSINGS

Mayonnaise	1 tablespoon	10g	0g	0g
Mustard	1 teaspoon	0g	0g	0g
Low-Sugar Ketchup	1 tablespoon	0g	0g	1g

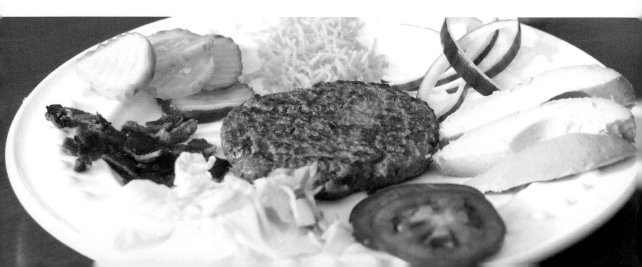

Salsa Chicken

*Dairy-free recipe with modifications

Ingredients

- 3 tablespoons olive oil, divided
- 2 cooked chicken breasts
- 1/2 (6-ounce) can tomato paste
- 1/4 cup chopped cilantro
- 1 tablespoon cumin
- 1 teaspoon cayenne pepper
- 1 teaspoon garlic powder
- 1 teaspoon onion powder

Directions

1. Heat 2 tablespoons of olive oil on skillet over medium-high heat.
2. Shred cooked chicken breasts and add to skillet.
3. Add in remaining 1 tablespoon olive oil, tomato paste, cilantro, cumin, cayenne pepper, garlic powder, and onion powder and cook until thoroughly heated.

Note: This dish is higher in protein than it is fat. To increase the fats, serve with half of an avocado, sour cream, and/or cheese.

Macros per serving: 13g F | 20g P | 1g NC

Makes 4 servings.

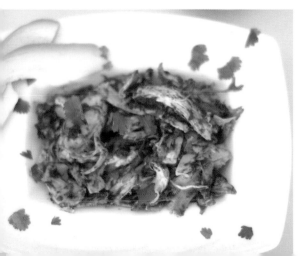

One-Pan Paprika Chicken and Veggies

*Dairy-free recipe with modifications

Ingredients

- 2 tablespoons paprika
- 1 teaspoon salt
- 1/2 teaspoon black pepper
- 1/2 teaspoon turmeric
- 1/2 teaspoon garlic powder
- 1 pound boneless and skinless chicken thighs
- 1 tablespoon avocado oil
- 1/2 large yellow onion, halved and sliced
- 1 cup cherry tomatoes
- 4 ounces baby spinach, finely chopped
- Fresh cilantro, finely chopped
- 2/3 cup full-fat coconut milk

Directions

1. Mix the paprika, salt, pepper, turmeric, and garlic powder together in a bowl, then add the chicken thighs and coat with the mixture.
2. In a pan over medium heat, heat avocado oil and add the chicken. Cook the chicken about 4 to 6 minutes on each side.
3. Add the onions and tomatoes, stir, and cook 5 to 6 more minutes. Mash the tomatoes to let out the juices in the pan.
4. Add in spinach, cilantro, and coconut milk and stir again.
5. Cook about 8 to 10 minutes more until chicken is fully cooked and enjoy!

Macros per serving: 18g F | 24g P | 5g NC

Makes 4 servings.

Creamy Chicken

Ingredients

12 ounces cream cheese

1 cup bone broth

2 pounds boneless, skinless chicken breast

2 (1-ounce) packets dry ranch seasoning mix

$1/2$ cup shredded Cheddar cheese

8 ounces cooked bacon, crumbled

Directions

1. Cut the cream cheese into large cubes.
2. Pour bone broth into an Instant Pot or a slow cooker.
3. Add in chicken and place the cream cheese and ranch seasoning mix over the chicken.
4. Turn your Instant Pot on high and cook for 12 minutes, then quick release. If using a slow cooker, turn on low for 5 hours.
5. Remove and shred the chicken.
6. Place the shredded chicken back into the pot and add cheese and bacon. Use them as toppings or mix all of them together.

Macros per serving: 20g F | 31g P | 5g NC

Makes 8 servings.

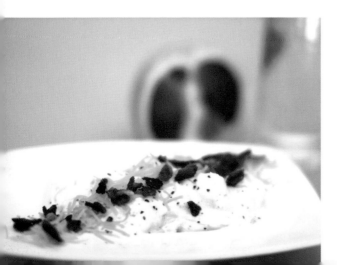

Pesto Chicken with Asparagus and Tomatoes

*Dairy-free recipe

Ingredients

1 pound boneless, skinless chicken thighs, sliced into strips

Salt and black pepper to taste

2 tablespoons olive oil

$1/3$ cup chopped sun-dried tomatoes, divided

1 pound asparagus, trimmed and cut in half

$1/4$ cup basil pesto

1 cup cherry tomatoes, halved

Directions

1. Season chicken with salt and pepper.
2. In a large pan over medium heat, cook the olive oil, chicken thighs, and half of the sun-dried tomatoes for 5 to 10 minutes. Stir to ensure chicken is evenly and fully cooked. Set chicken and tomatoes to the side. Keep oil in pan.
3. In the same pan on medium heat, add asparagus. Season with salt and pepper. Add remaining half of sun-dried tomatoes and cook 5 to 10 minutes. Ensure asparagus is fully cooked. Move asparagus to serving plate.
4. In the same pan on medium-low heat, cook chicken and pesto 1 to 2 minutes, then remove from heat. Add in cherry tomatoes and mix.
5. Place chicken and tomatoes with asparagus to serve.

Macros per serving: 32g F | 23g P | 8g NC

Makes 4 servings.

Chicken, Bacon, and Ranch Casserole

Ingredients

1 pound rotisserie chicken, chopped

1/2 pound bacon, cooked and chopped

1 cup shredded Cheddar cheese

4 large eggs

1/2 cup heavy whipping cream

1/2 cup full-fat ranch dressing

Directions

1. Preheat oven to 350 degrees.
2. Lightly coat a nonstick rimmed sheet with cooking spray.
3. Add chicken and bacon to the sheet and top with cheese.
4. In a bowl mix eggs, whipping cream, and dressing and pour over the meat and cheese.
5. Bake for 30 to 35 minutes.

Macros per serving: 29g F | 33g P | 4g NC

Makes 8 servings.

Cheesy BBQ Bacon Meatballs

Ingredients

1 pound 80/20 ground beef

1 pound ground sausage

1 large egg

1 small finely diced onion

1/2 cup shredded Cheddar cheese

2 pieces of cooked bacon, crumbled

1 teaspoon chili powder

1 teaspoon onion powder

1 teaspoon garlic powder

1 teaspoon salt

1 teaspoon black pepper

Sugar-free BBQ sauce

Directions

1. Preheat oven to 350 degrees.
2. Combine beef, sausage, egg, onion, cheese, bacon, chili powder, onion powder, garlic powder, salt, and pepper in a bowl. Form 12 equal-sized balls and place in a greased muffin tin.
3. Bake in oven for 40 minutes. Ten minutes prior to completion, drizzle sugar-free BBQ sauce on top.

Macros per serving: 30g F | 42g P | 1g NC

Makes 6 servings (2 balls per serving).

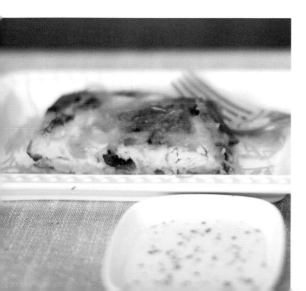

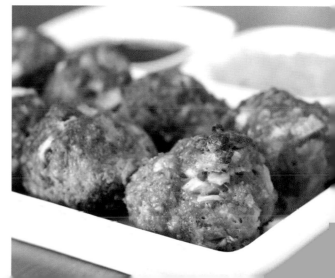

BBQ Bacon Meatloaf

Ingredients

- 1 pound $^{80}/20$ ground beef
- 1 pound ground sausage
- 1 large egg
- 1 small finely diced onion
- $^{1}/2$ cup shredded Cheddar cheese
- 2 pieces of cooked bacon, crumbled
- 1 teaspoon chili powder
- 1 teaspoon onion powder
- 1 teaspoon garlic powder
- 1 teaspoon salt
- 1 teaspoon black pepper
- Sugar-free BBQ sauce

Directions

1. Preheat oven to 350 degrees.
2. Combine beef, sausage, egg, onion, cheese, bacon, chili powder, onion powder, garlic powder, salt, and pepper in a bowl. Add beef mixture to a greased loaf pan.
3. Cook in oven for 60 minutes. Ten minutes prior to completion, drizzle sugar-free BBQ sauce on top.

Macros per serving: 30g F | 42g P | 1g NC

Makes 6 servings.

Low-Carb Meatloaf

Ingredients

- 1 $^{1}/2$ pounds ground beef
- 4 ounces crushed pork rinds
- $^{1}/4$ cup tomato sauce
- 1 large egg
- $^{1}/2$ cup grated Parmesan cheese
- $^{1}/4$ cup diced onion
- $^{1}/2$ teaspoon salt
- $^{1}/2$ teaspoon black pepper
- $^{1}/2$ teaspoon garlic salt
- $^{1}/2$ teaspoon onion powder

Directions

1. Preheat oven to 350 degrees.
2. In a medium bowl combine beef, pork rinds, tomato sauce, egg, Parmesan, onion, salt, pepper, garlic salt, and onion powder.
3. Add beef mixture to a greased loaf pan.
4. Bake for 1 hour, serve, and enjoy!

Macros per serving: 24g F | 25g P | 1g NC

Makes 8 servings.

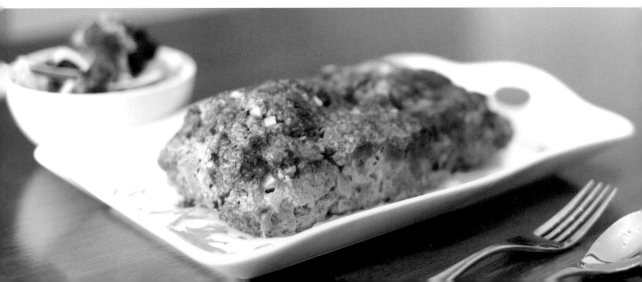

Beef and Broccoli Stir-Fry

*Dairy-free recipe with modifications

Ingredients

1 tablespoon butter (or vegan butter), divided

10 ounces ^{80}/20 ground beef

9 ounces broccoli, small florets and chopped stems

1 tablespoon mayonnaise

Salt and black pepper to taste

Directions

1. In a large pan over high heat, add ^{1}/2 tablespoon butter and brown the beef until almost fully cooked. Drain the fat.

2. Lower the heat and add remaining ^{1}/2 tablespoon butter. Add broccoli and cook for 4 minutes while stirring both the beef and broccoli together.

3. Mix in mayo, salt, and pepper. Enjoy!

Macros per serving: 34g F | 23g P | 5g NC

Makes 2 servings.

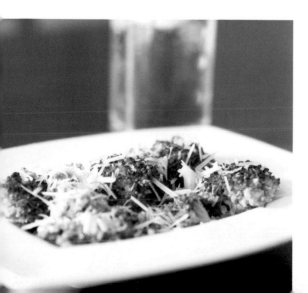

Spinach and Cheese–Stuffed Burgers

Ingredients

1 pound ^{80}/20 ground beef

1 teaspoon salt

^{3}/4 teaspoon black pepper

2 cups fresh baby spinach

^{1}/2 cup mozzarella shredded cheese (about 4 ounces)

2 tablespoons grated Parmesan cheese

Directions

1. In a medium bowl combine beef, salt, and pepper.

2. Scoop out the mixture (about ^{1}/3 cup) evenly to create eight patties.

3. Over medium-high heat, sauté the spinach in a pan until wilted. Drain excess liquid.

4. Chop the cooked spinach and place in a bowl. Add mozzarella and Parmesan, and mix together.

5. Scoop out this mixture (about ^{1}/4 cup) evenly and place in the center of four patties.

6. Place each of the four plain patties on top of the patty with mixture.

7. Round out all edges and slightly flatten into one full patty (4 total).

8. Grill or pan-fry on medium-high for 5 to 7 minutes on each side.

Macros per serving: 25g F | 25g P | 1g NC

Makes 4 servings.

Shrimp Fried Cauliflower Rice

*Dairy-free recipe with modifications

Ingredients

1 small onion, diced

4 tablespoons olive oil, divided

1/4 cup chopped broccoli

1 bag frozen riced cauliflower

Soy sauce (or coconut aminos) to taste

1 large egg

Garlic salt to taste

12 ounces cooked shrimp

Directions

1. In a skillet over medium-high heat, sauté the onions in 2 tablespoons of oil until they are tender. Add in broccoli and cook until soft.
2. Add cauliflower and cook until no longer frozen.
3. Add soy sauce.
4. Using half of the pan, scramble the egg. Once scrambled, combine it with the cauliflower mixture.
5. Add garlic salt.
6. In separate pan heat the remaining 2 tablespoons of oil in a skillet over medium-high heat.
7. Add shrimp and sauté until heated thoroughly, approximately 10 minutes. Add on top of riced cauliflower.

Macros per serving: 14g F | 21g P | 2g NC

Makes 4 servings.

Shrimp Ceviche

Ingredients

1 pound fresh shrimp, cooked, peeled, deveined, and chopped

1 avocado, chopped

1/2 cup cilantro, coarsely chopped

1 cucumber, peeled and chopped

1/3 cup fresh lime juice

1/2 cup red onion, chopped

1/2 cup tomatoes, chopped

1/2 teaspoon salt

1/4 teaspoon black pepper

1 tablespoon olive oil

Directions

1. Add shrimp, avocado, cilantro, cucumber, lime juice, onion, tomatoes, salt, pepper, and olive oil into a large bowl, then stir to combine well.
2. Serve immediately.
3. Option: Cover and place in refrigerator to sit and marinate for 1–4 hours before serving.

Macros per serving: 9g F | 28g P | 4g NC

Makes 4 servings.

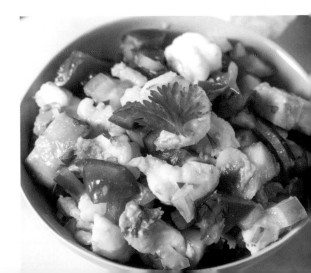

Chili Salmon and Sautéed Veggies

Ingredients

- 4 tablespoons butter
- 2 teaspoons chili paste
- 1 pound wild-caught salmon
- 1 pound asparagus, chopped to 4-inch lengths
- Salt and black pepper to taste
- 4 ounces cherry tomatoes, halved
- 2 tablespoons olive oil, divided
- 2 tablespoons thyme (dried or fresh)
- 1 ounce almonds, sliced (optional)

Directions

1. In a pan over medium heat, melt butter fully but don't allow it to burn. Set to the side and keep warm.
2. In a small bowl mix chili paste with 2 tablespoons water and spread over the salmon. Add salt and pepper to your liking.
3. In a large pan over medium-high heat, add 1 tablespoon olive oil and cook the salmon for several minutes on both sides.
4. Add remaining 1 tablespoon olive oil to the pan and sauté the asparagus and tomatoes for 2 to 3 minutes.
5. Serve salmon with sautéed veggies and top with thyme, almonds, and melted butter.

Macros per serving: 26g F | 25g P | 4g NC

Makes 4 servings.

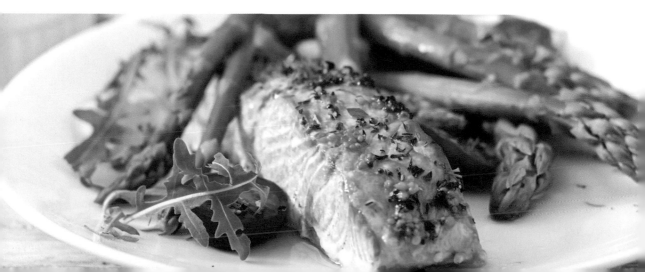

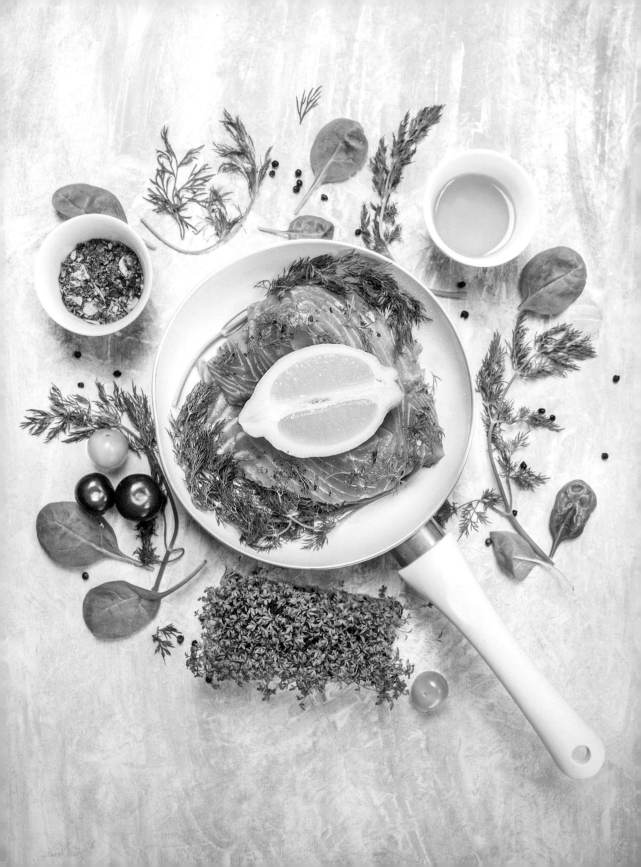

SIDES

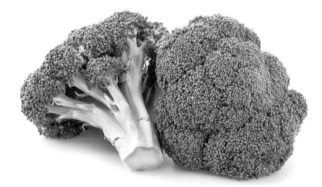

90-Second Bread

Ingredients

1 $\frac{1}{4}$ tablespoons butter, softened, divided

1 large egg

1 tablespoon coconut flour

1 teaspoon sour cream

$\frac{1}{4}$ teaspoon baking powder

1 tablespoon shredded Cheddar cheese

Directions

1. Add $\frac{1}{4}$ tablespoon butter, egg, coconut flour, sour cream, baking powder, and cheese to a microwave-safe bowl and mix together.
2. Heat mixture for 90 seconds in microwave, remove, and let sit until cool.
3. Melt 1 tablespoon of butter on the stove.
4. Cut the bread in half and heat each side in a skillet until firm.

Macros per serving: 24g F | 9g P | 3g NC

Makes 1 serving.

Fried Green Beans

*Dairy-free recipe

Ingredients

4 cups fresh green beans

2 tablespoons olive or avocado oil

2 teaspoons minced garlic

Salt and black pepper to taste

$\frac{1}{2}$ teaspoon cayenne pepper

$\frac{1}{2}$ teaspoon onion powder

$\frac{1}{2}$ teaspoon garlic salt

1 tablespoon liquid aminos, coconut aminos, or soy sauce

Directions

1. Trim ends off green beans and place in a microwave-safe bowl.
2. Microwave on high for 9 minutes to soften.
3. In a skillet heat oil over medium-high heat. Add garlic and sauté until fragrant.
4. Add green beans, salt, pepper, cayenne, and onion powder and sauté for 4 to 5 minutes.
5. Just before removing from heat, add in liquid aminos and sauté an additional 1 to 2 minutes.

Macros per serving: 7g F | 1g P | 2g NC

Makes 4 servings.

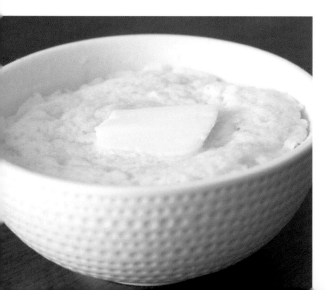

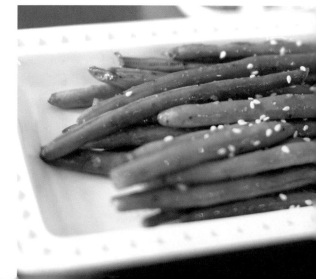

Cauli-Mash

Ingredients

- 1 (12-ounce) bag of riced cauliflower or cauliflower florets
- 2 tablespoons butter
- 4 tablespoons heavy whipping cream
- Salt and black pepper to taste

Directions

1. Pierce bag of cauliflower and microwave on high for 4 minutes. Cauliflower should be soft.
2. Once thoroughly heated, add cauliflower, butter, whipping cream, salt, and pepper into a food processor and blend until thoroughly combined. If no food processer is available, a traditional blender can be used.
3. Serve alongside one of your favorite main courses.

Macros per serving: 12g F | 2g P | 3g NC

Makes 4 servings.

Zesty Broccoli

*Dairy-free recipe

Ingredients

- 1 (10-ounce) bag of broccoli (fresh or frozen)
- 2 tablespoons of olive oil
- 1 tablespoon of liquid aminos, coconut aminos, or soy sauce
- $1/2$ teaspoon salt
- $1/2$ teaspoon black pepper
- $1/2$ teaspoon garlic powder
- $1/2$ teaspoon onion powder

Directions

1. Preheat oven to 425 degrees.
2. In a large resealable baggie or bowl, combine broccoli, olive oil, aminos, salt, pepper, garlic powder, and onion powder and mix.
3. Spread broccoli mixture evenly on a foil-lined baking sheet.
4. Cook in oven for 30 minutes (fresh) or 40 minutes (frozen). Broccoli should be tender and browning around the edges.

Macros per serving: 7g F | 2g P | 3g NC

Makes 4 servings.

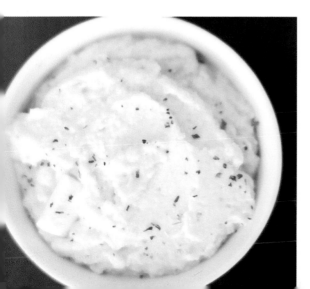

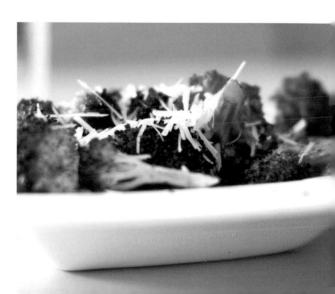

Cauliflower Mac-n-Cheese

Ingredients

- 1 large head of cauliflower, cut into small pieces
- 1 cup heavy cream
- 1 teaspoon Dijon mustard
- 2 ounces cream cheese, cut into small pieces
- 2 cups shredded Cheddar cheese, divided, plus 1/2 cup for topping
- Salt and black pepper to taste
- 1/2 teaspoon garlic powder

Directions

1. Preheat oven to 375 degrees.
2. In a large pot bring water to a boil. Add in cauliflower and cook for 5 minutes. The cauliflower should be somewhat tender, but not fully cooked.
3. Drain cauliflower and use paper towels to pat dry and absorb excess liquid.
4. Spray 8 x 8-inch baking dish with cooking spray. Transfer cauliflower to baking dish.
5. Bring the cream and mustard to a simmer over medium-low heat in a pan and add the cream cheese. Stir in 1 1/2 cups of shredded Cheddar, salt, pepper, and garlic powder and whisk until completely melted.
6. Remove from heat and pour over cauliflower. Use a spoon to mix together.
7. Top the dish with remaining 1/2 cup of shredded Cheddar and cook in oven for 15 minutes.

Tip: Broiling for the last 2 minutes gives a nice browned and bubbly topping.

Macros per serving: 20g F | 8g P | 4g NC

Makes 9 servings.

Creamed Spinach

Ingredients

- 1 (16-ounce) package of fresh spinach
- 2 tablespoons butter
- 1 teaspoon minced garlic
- 2 ounces cream cheese
- 1/2 cup heavy cream
- 1/4 cup shredded Parmesan cheese
- 1/2 teaspoon onion powder
- Salt and black pepper to taste

Directions

1. Chop the fresh spinach into small pieces.
2. In a large skillet over medium heat, sauté butter and garlic. Mix in spinach and cook until spinach is wilted. Remove from heat.
3. In a separate pan mix cream cheese, heavy cream, and Parmesan together. Cook over medium-high heat, stirring frequently, until the entire mixture is melted.
4. Add onion powder, salt, and pepper.
5. Combine the melted cheese sauce to the spinach pan.

Macros per serving: 16g F | 4g P | 2g NC

Makes 6 servings.

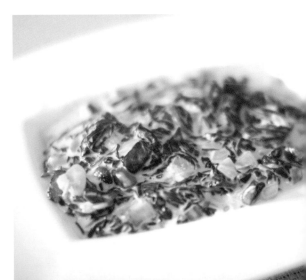

DESSERTS AND SNACKS

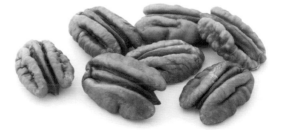

Cinnamon Sugar Tortilla

*Dairy-free recipe with modifications

Ingredients

- 1 tablespoon butter (or vegan butter)
- 1 small low-carb tortilla
- 1 tablespoon granulated Swerve or stevia
- 1 teaspoon ground cinnamon

Directions

1. In a large skillet melt butter over medium-high heat.
2. Add tortilla and cook for 30 seconds on each side.
3. Top with $1/2$ tablespoon of Swerve and $1/2$ teaspoon of cinnamon on each side, continuously flipping over heat.
4. Remove from heat and roll up. For extra fat, an extra $1/2$ tablespoon of butter can be added as a topping.

Macros per serving: 13g F | 3g P | 4.5g NC

Makes 1 serving.

Keto Candied Pecans

*Dairy-free recipe with modifications

Ingredients

- 3 tablespoons butter (or vegan butter)
- 1 cup whole pecans
- 3 tablespoons granulated Swerve or stevia
- 1 tablespoon ground cinnamon

Directions

1. In a medium-sized pan over medium-high heat, melt butter.
2. Stir in pecans, Swerve or stevia, and cinnamon.
3. Continuously stirring, cook for 5 minutes until thoroughly coated.
4. Remove from heat and allow to cool for 5 minutes.
5. Add additional 1 tablespoon of Swerve on top and stir to coat.

Macros per serving: 14g F | 1g P | 5g NC

Makes 8 servings.

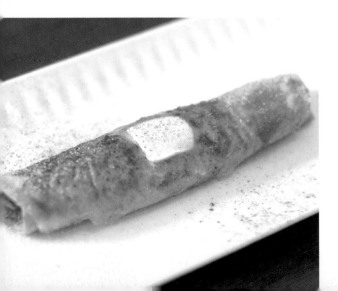

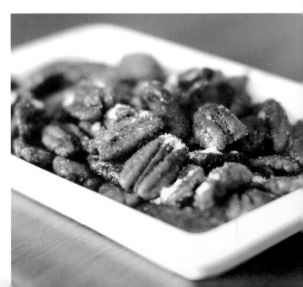

Keto Chocolate Chip Cookies

Ingredients

1 cup almond flour

$1/3$ cup coconut flour

1 tablespoon xanthan gum

$1/2$ teaspoon baking soda

$1/4$ teaspoon baking powder

$1/4$ teaspoon salt

$1/3$ cup butter (or vegan butter), softened

$1/2$ cup erythritol (Swerve)

1 teaspoon pure vanilla extract

2 large eggs

$1/3$ cup Stevia-sweetened chocolate chips

Directions

1. Preheat oven to 350 degrees.
2. In a large bowl combine almond flour, coconut flour, xanthan gum, baking soda, baking powder, and salt.
3. In a separate bowl mix together butter, erythritol, and vanilla until well combined. Add in eggs and mix until smooth.
4. Combine the butter mixture and the flour mixture and stir with a spoon. This should be a dough consistency. If not, continue to add 1 tablespoon of almond flour until a dough consistency is reached.
5. Fold in chocolate chips and refrigerate for 30 minutes.
6. Roll the dough into 16 separate balls and place on a greased cookie sheet. Flatten slightly with the back of a spoon or spatula.
7. Cook in oven for 8 to 10 minutes or until the bottoms are slightly browned.
8. Remove from oven and allow the cookies to rest on the heated cookie sheet for 20 minutes.

Macros per serving: 10g F | 3g P | 2g NC

Makes 16 servings.

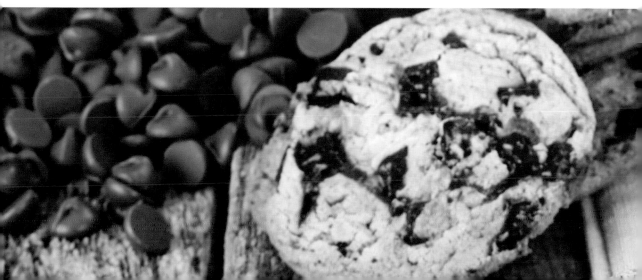

Peanut Butter Bliss

*Dairy-free recipe with modifications

Ingredients

- 8 ounces peanut butter
- $1/3$ cup powdered erythritol (Swerve)
- 2 tablespoons butter (or vegan butter), melted

Directions

1. Put peanut butter, erythritol, and butter in a bowl.
2. Mix well and enjoy!

Macros per serving: 17g F | 5.5g P | 5g NC

Makes 8 servings.

Chocolate Peanut Butter Bliss

*Dairy-free recipe with modifications

Ingredients

- 8 ounces peanut butter
- $1/3$ cup powdered erythritol (Swerve)
- $1/4$ cup cocoa powder, unsweetened
- 3 tablespoons butter (or vegan butter), melted

Directions

1. Put peanut butter, erythritol, cocoa powder, and butter in a bowl.
2. Mix well and enjoy!

Macros per serving: 18g F | 7g P | 5.5g NC

Makes 8 servings.

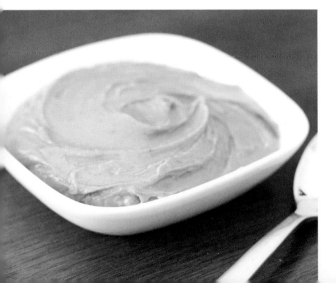

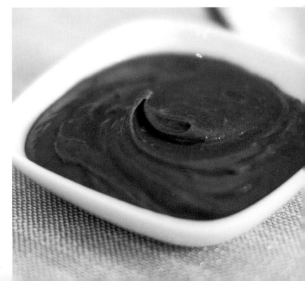

Cookie Dough Fat Bomb

Ingredients

- 1 (8-ounce) package cream cheese, softened
- 3 tablespoons butter, softened
- 6 tablespoons all-natural peanut butter (no sugar added)
- 1 tablespoon pure vanilla extract
- 1/3 cup powdered erythritol (Swerve)
- 1/3 cup dark chocolate chips (Lily's if budget allows!)

Directions

1. Mix cream cheese, butter, peanut butter, vanilla, and erythritol together in the bowl of a mixer until well combined.
2. Fold in chocolate chips.
3. Scoop mixture into 12 balls on a cookie sheet and freeze for 1 hour.
4. Cookie dough balls can be stored in the freezer. Remove from freezer 20 minutes prior to eating in order to thaw.

Macros per serving: 16g F | 2.5g P | 4g NC

Makes 12 servings.

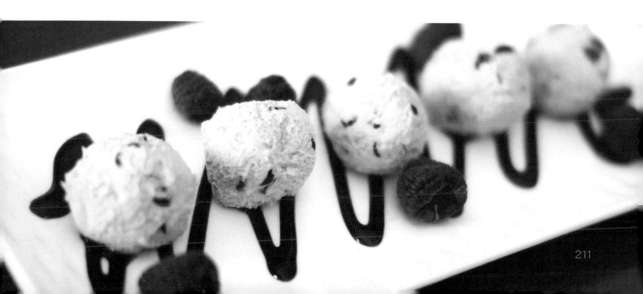

Snacks

Macadamia Nuts
1 ounce
21g F | 2g P | 1g NC

Almonds
1 ounce
15g F | 7g P | 4g NC

Celery and Peanut Butter
2 stalks and 2 tablespoons
16g F | 7g P | 4g NC

Pork Rinds
2 ounces
5g F | 8g P | 0g NC

Cheese Stick
1 stick
6g F | 7g P | 1g NC

Tuna Creations
1 package
1g F | 15g P | 1g NC

Cheese Whisps
1 ounce
11g F | 13g P | 1g NC

Prosciutto
1 ounce
3g F | 8g P | 1g NC

Flackers, Sea Salt
10 crackers
12g F | 6g P | 1g NC

Wholly Guacamole
2 ounces
9g F | 1g P | 2g NC

Sliced Cucumber
1 ounce
0g F | 0g P | 1g NC

Kirkland Roasted Seaweed
1 package
8g F | 5g P | 0g NC

Pickles
6 slices
0g F | 0g P | 1g NC

Olives
8 pieces
5g F | 0g P | 0g NC

Jimmy Dean Bacon Scramblers
1 package
21g F | 24g P | 2g NC

Starbucks Egg Bites
1 order
22g F | 19g P | 9g NC

VEGAN RECIPES

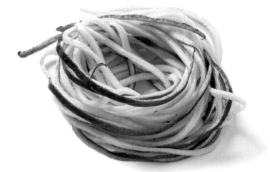

Vanilla Overnight "Oats"

Ingredients

- 1 cup full-fat coconut milk, divided
- 2 tablespoons chia seeds
- $1/4$ cup hemp hearts
- 2 teaspoons of Swerve or stevia (granular)
- $1/2$ teaspoon pure vanilla extract
- $1/4$ teaspoon salt
- 10 almonds for topping

Directions

1. Add $2/3$ cup coconut milk, chia seeds, hemp hearts, Swerve or stevia, vanilla, and salt to a large container and mix. Cover the container and allow to chill in the fridge for no less than 8 hours.
2. After 8 hours, top your "oats" with remaining $1/3$ cup coconut milk and almonds.

Macros per serving: 36g F | 13g P | 4g NC

Makes 2 servings.

Breakfast Shake

Ingredients

- 1 scoop vegan protein powder (OWYN is a great brand)
- 1 cup full-fat coconut milk
- 2 teaspoons stevia

Directions

1. Add protein powder, coconut milk, and stevia to a shaker or mixer.
2. Shake or mix well to combine thoroughly.

Macros per serving: 36g F | 12g P | 8g NC

Makes 1 serving.

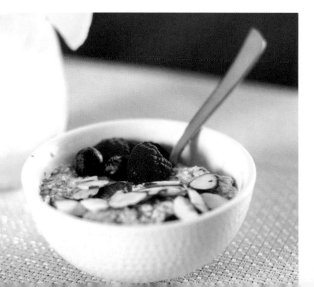

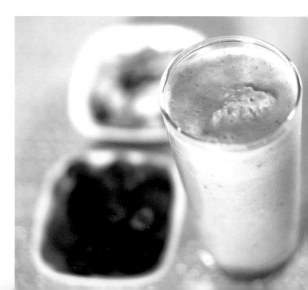

Breakfast Scramble

Ingredients

1 package firm tofu

3 tablespoons avocado or olive oil

2 tablespoons onion, chopped

$1/2$ teaspoon garlic powder

$1/2$ teaspoon turmeric

Salt and black pepper to taste

2 tablespoons nutritional yeast

1 cup fresh spinach

4 grape tomatoes

3 ounces vegan shredded Cheddar cheese

2 avocados

Directions

1. Squeeze any water out of tofu using a paper towel.

2. In a skillet over medium-high heat, add oil and sauté onions until they become translucent.

3. Add block of tofu and garlic powder, turmeric, salt, and pepper. Mash until tofu develops a scrambled egg consistency.

4. Continue to cook so that there is no excess liquid, then add yeast, spinach, tomatoes, and cheese.

5. Cook until cheese has melted.

6. Serve with half an avocado.

Macros per serving: 32g F | 13g P | 7g NC

Makes 4 servings.

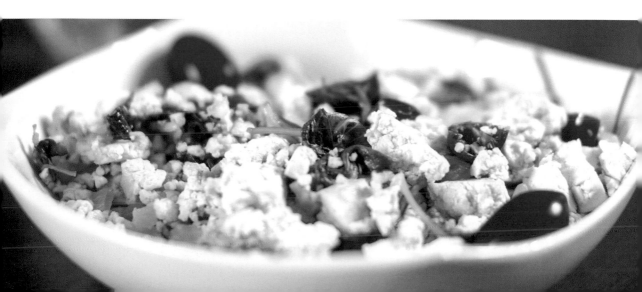

Cashew Crack Slaw

Ingredients

3 tablespoons avocado or olive oil

1/2 small onion, diced

1 bell pepper, finely diced

1 cup mushrooms, sliced

1 cup cashews, chopped or whole

4 cups shredded cabbage

1/4 cup liquid aminos, coconut aminos, or soy sauce

Salt and black pepper to taste

Directions

1. In a large pan on medium-high heat, add the oil and onions and stir-fry for 2 to 3 minutes.
2. Add peppers, mushrooms, and cashews and stir-fry an additional 5 minutes.
3. Next add cabbage and aminos. Mix well and cook until cabbage becomes wilted. Then add salt and pepper.

Macros per serving: 23g F | 7g P | 11g NC

Makes 3 servings.

Creamy Zucchini Pasta

Ingredients

1 avocado

1 teaspoon garlic

1/2 cup fresh basil leaves

1 tablespoon lime juice

3 tablespoons avocado or olive oil, divided

Water, as needed

2 zucchinis, spiralized

Salt and black pepper to taste

Directions

1. In a food processor blend avocado, garlic, basil, and lime juice until smooth. Slowly stir in 2 tablespoons of oil. Add water to reach a sauce-like consistency.
2. In a pan over medium-high heat, sauté zucchini noodles in the remaining 1 tablespoon oil until tender.
3. Remove from heat and drain any excess liquid. Add avocado dressing and toss before serving.

Macros per serving: 31g F | 3g P | 3g NC

Makes 2 servings.

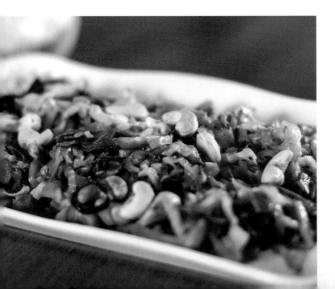

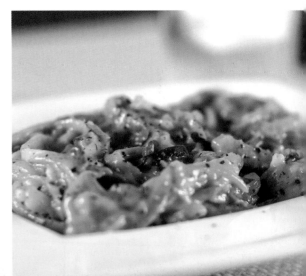

Mexican Cauliflower Rice

Ingredients

3 cups cauliflower florets

3 tablespoons avocado or olive oil

1/2 onion, small diced

1 jalapeño, chopped

3 teaspoons minced garlic

1 tablespoon fresh cilantro, chopped

1/2 teaspoon chili powder

1/2 teaspoon cumin

Salt and black pepper to taste

1 tomato, medium diced

1/2 cup diced bell pepper

1 1/2 avocados

Directions

1. Use a food processer to chop cauliflower until it resembles rice.

2. In a large pan over medium heat, add oil, onions, jalapeño, and garlic. Cook until garlic is fragrant.

3. Add chili powder, cumin, salt, and tomato and cook about 3 minutes.

4. Add in bell pepper and cauliflower rice and pan-fry for 3 to 4 minutes until rice is tender.

5. Top with cilantro and serve with half an avocado.

Macros per serving: 31g F | 6g P | 9g NC

Makes 3 servings.

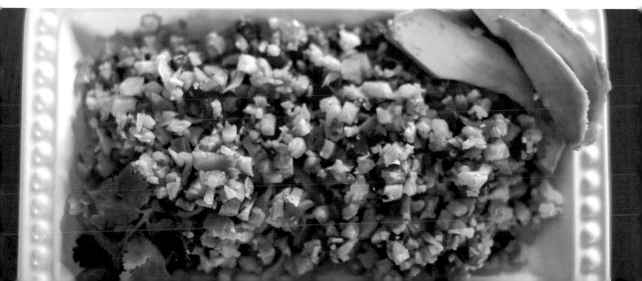

VEGAN STIR-FRY BOWLS

PROTEIN

Food Item	Quantity	Fat	Protein	Net Carbs
Chia Seeds	1/4 cup	12g	7g	3g
Edamame	1/2 cup	4g	9g	3g
Hemp Hearts	1/4 cup	17g	13g	0g
Seitan	3 ounces	2g	21g	3g
Tofu	4 ounces	3g	8g	3g

FATS

Food Item	Quantity	Fat	Protein	Net Carbs
Avocados	1/2	21g	3g	2g
Avocado or Olive Oil	1 tablespoon	14g	0g	0g
Vegan Butter	1 tablespoon	11g	0g	0g

VEGGIES

Food Item	Quantity	Fat	Protein	Net Carbs
Baby Spinach	1/2 cup	0g	0g	0g
Bell Peppers	1/2 cup	0g	1g	2g
Broccoli	1/2 cup	0g	1g	2g
Brussels Sprouts	1/2 cup	0g	1g	2g
Mushrooms	1/4 cup	0g	0g	0g
Onions	2 tablespoons	0g	0g	2g

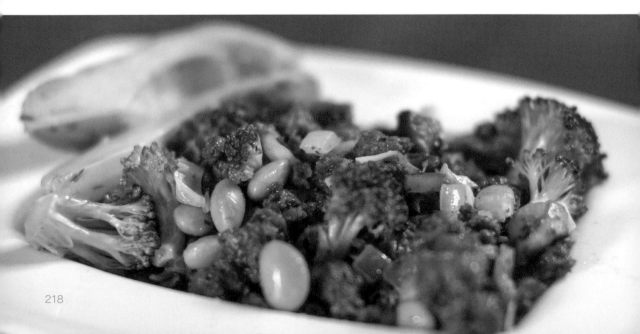

VEGAN SALAD BOWL

PROTEIN

Food Item	Quantity	Fat	Protein	Net Carbs
Chia Seeds	1/4 cup	12g	7g	3g
Edamame	1/2 cup	4g	9g	3g
Hemp Hearts	1/4 cup	17g	13g	0g
Seitan	3 ounces	2g	21g	3g
Tofu	4 ounces	3g	8g	3g

FATS

Avocados	1/2	21g	3g	2g
Almonds	1 ounce	14g	0g	0g
Pumpkin Seeds	1/4 cup	14g	9g	2g

VEGGIES

Baby Spinach	1/2 cup	0g	0g	0g
Lettuce	2 cups	0g	0g	2g
Romaine	2 cups	0g	1g	2g
Bell Peppers	1/2 cup	0g	1g	2g
Broccoli	1/2 cup	0g	1g	2g
Mushrooms	1/4 cup	0g	0g	2g
Onions	2 tablespoons	0g	0g	2g
Tomatoes	1/3 cup	0g	1g	2g

DRESSINGS

Annie's Goddess	2 tablespoons	12g	1g	2g
Balsamic Vinaigrette	2 tablespoons	10g	0g	3g
Oil and Vinegar	2 tablespoons	18g	0g	0g
Vegan Caesar	2 tablespoons	7g	0g	1g
Vegan Ranch	2 tablespoons	15g	0g	1g

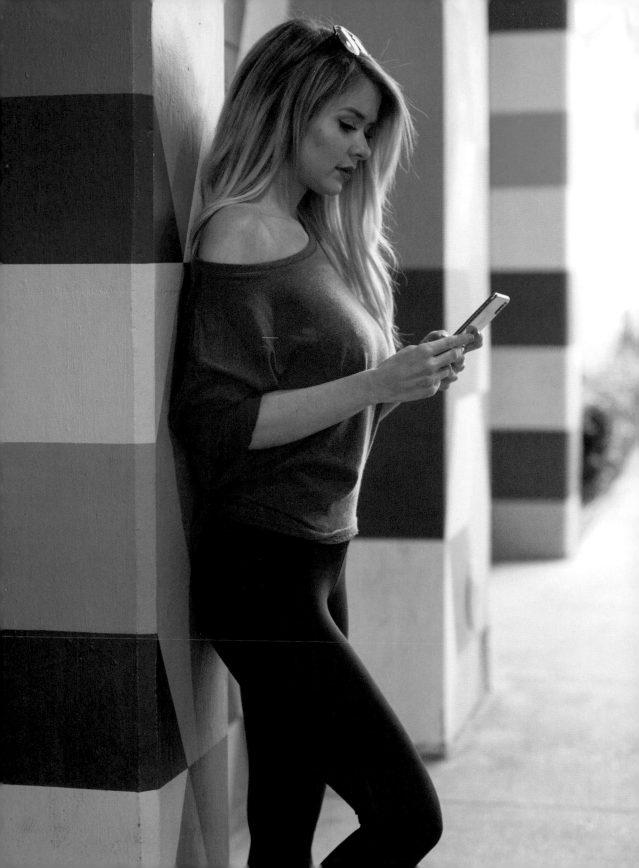

RESTAURANT OPTIONS

In general, fast food and restaurants are never going to be the healthiest options, because the vast majority of them use less-healthy fats to cook their food in. Additionally, it can be difficult to accurately track what you are consuming. However, sometimes life brings us to the drive-through. I would rather show you what the best options are to stick to this diet style than leave you wondering what to select.

The overall idea is to give you an idea of what kinds of foods make the best options. I've included a list of popular chain restaurants along with some general types of cuisines that fit many restaurant options nation-wide. You may not have the exact same steak restaurant close to your home, but you can use the suggestions below to help guide your decisions at a similar place.

Arby's

Grand Turkey Club

Order a Grand Turkey Club with no bun. Instead of fries, opt for a side salad with ranch or Caesar dressing. Or order a bunless sandwich à la carte.

20g F | 26g P | 4g NC (entrée only)

Roast Beef Gyro

Order a Roast Beef Gyro with no flatbread. Instead of fries, opt for a side salad with ranch or Caesar dressing. Or order the entrée à la carte.

23g F | 17g P | 4g NC

Buffalo Wild Wings

Wings and Tenders

While chicken wings and naked tenders are great from a low-carb perspective, they are high in protein.

Naked Wings (16gF | 35gP | 0gNC)
Naked Tenders, 3-piece (0gF | 37gP | 0gNC)

Chicken Caesar Salad

Order without croutons or garlic bread.

50g F | 42g P | 8g NC

Grilled Chicken Santa Fe Salad

Order without corn, tortillas, or chips and with southwestern ranch dressing.

79g F | 49g P | 12g NC

Garden Chicken Salad

Order without the croutons or bread and with blue cheese or ranch dressing.

47g F | 41g P | 12g NC

BYOB (Build Your Own Burger)

All of the options below are keto-friendly. Order by selecting your protein, cheese, and toppings.

Protein Base:

Hamburger patty (32g F | 30g P | 0g NC)
Grilled chicken breast (27g F | 29g P | 1g NC)

Cheese:

American cheese (5g F | 3g P | 2g NC)
Cheddar jack cheese (4.5g F | 3g P | 1g NC)
Cheddar cheese (7g F | 5g P | 0g NC)
Swiss cheese (4g F | 4g P | 0g NC)
Pepper jack cheese (6g F | 4g P | 0g NC)

Toppings:

Bacon slices (8g F | 8g P | 0g NC)

Beer-braised mushrooms (0g F | 2g P | 4g NC)

Avocado (15g F | 2g P | 2g NC)

Mayonnaise (10g F | 0g P | 0g NC)

Mustard (0g F | 0g P | 0g NC)

Burger King

Breakfast Sausage, Egg, and Cheese Sandwich

Order a "Croissan'wich" sausage, egg, and cheese sandwich. Before eating, remove the bun.

25g F | 16g P | 1g NC

Breakfast Platter

Ask for two sausage patties and two eggs à la carte.

Sausage and Eggs (36g F | 24g P | 5g NC)

Bunless Cheeseburgers

Order two single cheeseburgers with no bun. Cheeseburgers come with pickles and ketchup and will be served on a platter. Add mayo for additional fat.

Cheeseburgers (18g F | 20g P | 4g NC)

Chicken Club Salad

Order a Chicken Club Salad without croutons.

35g F | 35g P | 9g NC

Chick-fil-A

Thank goodness for Chick-fil-A! Please pay very close attention to the macros for various sauces. I have included a sauce list below to help you find the best option for you.

Sausage, Egg, and Cheese Biscuit

Order a sausage, egg, and cheese biscuit and throw away the biscuit.

40g F | 20g P | 4g NC (sandwich only)

8-Count Chicken Nuggets

Original (12g F | 18g P | 8g NC)
Grilled (3g F | 25g P | 2g NC)

Side Salad

Order a side salad in place of fries. Use the dressing list below to select a dressing that will keep you on track for your daily macro goal.

5g F | 5g P | 3g NC

Dressings and Sauces

Garlic and Herb Ranch Dressing (29g F | 1g P | 2g NC)

Avocado and Lime Ranch Dressing (32g F | 1g P | 3g NC)

Chick-fil-A Sauce (13g F | 0g P | 6g NC)

Garlic and Herb Ranch Sauce (14g F | 0g P | 1g NC)

Zesty Buffalo Sauce (4.5g F | 0g P | 1g NC)

Chili's

Appetizers

Buffalo Wings (65g F | 62g P | 5g NC)

Cup of Chili (14g F | 14g P | 6g NC)

Fresco Salad (10g F | 3g P | 6g NC)

Bunless Burgers

Guacamole Burger (65g F | 50g P | 5g NC)

Sunrise Burger (70g F | 62g P | 3g NC)

Oldtimer Burger (51g F | 50g P | 2g NC)

Ribs and Steaks

Classic Sirloin with Avocado and Broccoli (43g F | 48g P | 2g NC)

Classic Ribeye (64g F | 81g P | 1g NC)

Fajitas

Steak (15g F | 26g P | 0g NC)

Chicken (3.5g F | 28g P | 0g NC)

Shrimp (2g F | 11g P | 1g NC)

Chipotle

Christine's Chipotle Bowl

Order a bowl with chicken, veggies, sour cream, cheese, and guacamole. Top with Sriracha or Tabasco for extra spice.

46g F | 43g P | 9g NC

Build Your Own Bowl (BYOB)
Protein:

Chicken (7g F | 32g P | 0g NC)

Steak (6g F | 21g P | 1g NC)

Carnitas (12g F | 23g P | 0g NC)

Barbacoa (7g F | 24g P | 2g NC)

Chorizo (18g F | 32g P | 2g NC)

Toppings:

Fajita veggies (0g F | 1g P | 4g NC)

Sour cream (9g F | 2g P | 2g NC)

Cheese (8g F | 6g P | 1g NC)

Guacamole (22g F | 2g P | 2g NC)

Romaine lettuce (0g F | 0g P | 0g NC)

Any salsa (0g F | 0g P | 4g NC)

Things to Avoid:

- Tortillas
- Sofritas
- Rice
- Beans

- Corn
- Salad dressings
- Chips

Five Guys

Five Guys has some great keto-friendly options. When I order, I always go for a burger bowl (or lettuce wrap) and add toppings.

Christine's Favorite Burger Bowl

Order the bacon cheeseburger bowl and top with mayo, onions, and jalapeños.

41g F | 24g P | 2g NC

BYOBB (Build Your Own Burger Bowl)

All of the options below are keto-friendly. Order by selecting your protein, toppings, and sauces.

Protein Base:

Hamburger patty (17g F | 16g P | 0g NC)

Toppings:

Cheese (6g F | 4g P | 0g NC)

Bacon (7g F | 4g P | 0g NC)

Green peppers (0g F | 0g P | 1g NC)

Grilled mushrooms (0g F | 0g P | 1g NC)

Jalapeños (0g F | 0g P | 0g NC)

Pickles (0g F | 0g P | 1g NC)

Onions (0g F | 0g P | 2g NC)

Grilled onions (0g F | 0g P | 2g NC)

Tomatoes (0g F | 0g P | 2g NC)

Relish (0g F | 0g P | 3g NC)

Mayonnaise (11g F | 0g P | 0g NC)

Mustard (0g F | 0g P | 0g NC)

IHOP

À la Carte Options

Fried eggs (12g F | 13g P | 1g NC)

Hard/soft-boiled eggs (11g F | 13g P | 1g NC)

Poached eggs (8g F | 11g P | 1g NC)

Scrambled eggs (17g F | 15g P | 2g NC)

Bacon (12g F | 14g P | 2g NC)

Sausage links (34g F | 12g P | 1g NC)

Avocado (7g F | 1g P | 1g NC)

In-N-Out Burger

Cheeseburger "Protein Style"

Order a cheeseburger and ask for it to be "protein style." This burger comes with meat, cheese, tomato, and mayo spread.

25g F | 18g P | 8g NC (entrée only)

Double-Double "Protein Style"

Order a Double-Double and ask for it to be "protein style." This burger is double meat and double cheese, served in a lettuce wrap.

40g F | 33g P | 8g NC (entrée only)

Jimmy John's

Jimmy John's has amazing keto options because all of their sandwiches can be turned into an "Unwich," which is a sandwich in a lettuce wrap!

Turkey, Ham, and Provolone Unwich (28g F | 33g P | 6g NC)

Turkey, Provolone, and Avocado Unwich (38g F | 31g P | 6g NC)

Veggie Club Unwich (55g F | 33g P | 7g NC)

Turkey and Roast Beef Unwich (21g F | 30g P | 3g NC)

Tuna Salad and Provolone Unwich (40g F | 27g P | 7g NC)

Sliced Turkey and Bacon Unwich (25g F | 21g P | 3g NC)

Ultimate Ham BLT Unwich (26g F | 18g P | 4g NC)

Roast Beef, Ham, and Provolone Unwich (31g F | 35g P | 5g NC)

Big Italian Unwich (44g F | 33g P | 8g NC)

Ham and Provolone Unwich (28g F | 19g P | 5g NC)

Original Roast Beef Unwich (20g F | 16g P | 2g NC)

Tuna Salad Unwich (22g F | 11g P | 5g NC)

Turkey Unwich (18g F | 14g P | 3g NC)

Perfect Italian Unwich (25g F | 22g P | 6g NC)

McDonald's

Egg McMuffin

Order an à la carte Egg McMuffin with no bun.

11g F | 12g P | 3g NC (entrée only)

Sausage, Egg, and Cheese à la Carte

Order one piece of sausage, one round egg, and one slice of cheese.

27g F | 12g P | 4g NC (entrée only)

Bacon McDouble

Order one Bacon McDouble with no bun.

23g F | 28g P | 6g NC (entrée only)

Panda Express

Grilled Teriyaki Chicken

Order the Grilled Teriyaki Chicken, entrée only, with no sides.

13g F | 36g P | 8g NC (entrée only)

String Bean Chicken Breast

Order the String Bean Chicken Breast, entrée only, with no sides.

9g F | 14g P | 9g NC (entrée only)

Mushroom Chicken

Order the Mushroom Chicken, entrée only, with no sides.

14g F | 12g P | 10g NC (entrée only)

Fortune Cookie

Fortune cookies probably aren't a good diet food, but at 1.5 net carbs, they are definitely sweet-tooth crushers that won't hurt your waistline.

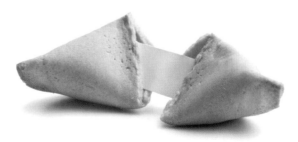

Panera Bread

Asian Sesame Salad with Chicken (Half)

Order the half portion of the Asian Sesame Salad with chicken and ask for no toasted chips

11g F | 16g P | 8g NC (entrée only).

Chicken Caesar Salad (Half)

Order the half portion of the Chicken Caesar Salad.

14g F | 17g P | 7g NC (entrée only).

Greek Salad (Whole)

Order the whole portion of the Greek Salad.

36g F | 6g P | 7g NC (entrée only).

Green Goddess Cobb Salad with Chicken (Half)

Order the half portion of the Green Goddess Cobb Salad with chicken.

16g F | 21g P | 8g NC (entrée only).

Order any of the following items à la carte to build your breakfast:

Over-easy eggs (6g F | 7g P | 2g NC)

Scrambled eggs (7g F | 8g P | 1g NC)

Sausage (13g F | 9g P | 1g NC)

Bacon (5g F | 5g P | 1g NC)

Avocado (4g F | 1g P | 0g NC)

Starbucks

Christine's Pink Drink

Order a grande iced passion fruit tea, no water, add extra heavy whipping cream, no classic syrup, and three stevia.

35g F | 0g P | 4g NC

Bacon Egg Bites

Order one order of the Bacon Egg Bites, which comes with two pieces.

22g F | 19g P | 9g NC

Hot Short Keto Latte

Order a short americano, $3/4$ water, and $1/4$ heavy whipping cream with foam on top.

5.5g F | 0g P | 1g NC

Hot Short Keto Mocha

Order a short mocha with sugar-free mocha syrup, and replace milk with $1/2$ heavy whipping cream and $1/2$ water.

5g F | 0g P | 1g NC

Hot Short Keto Flat White

Order a short flat white and replace steamed milk with $1/2$ heavy whipping cream and $1/2$ water (steamed).

5g F | 0g P | 1g NC

Hot Short Keto Chai Tea Latte

Order a short chai tea latte with 2 chai-brewed tea bags (not concentrate), 2 shots of heavy whipping cream, and 2 pumps of sugar-free cinnamon dolce.

5.5g F | 0g P | 1g NC

Hot Keto Peppermint Mocha

Order a grande americano, 2 shots of heavy whipping cream, 1 pump of peppermint syrup, and 4 pumps of sugar-free mocha.

5.5g F | 0g P | 5g NC

Iced Mocha

Order a grande cold foam cold brew. Ask for one pump of skinny mocha and two pumps of sugar-free vanilla. Ask for cold foam to be made with sugar-free vanilla. Ask for light heavy whipping cream.

8g F | 1g P | 5g NC

Green Tea

Order a venti green tea, no classic syrup, and add 4 stevia.

0g F | 0g P | 0g NC

Iced Espresso

Order an iced doppio espresso, add 4 stevia and a splash of heavy whipping cream.

10g F | 0g P | 4g NC

Subway

Subway Salads

Subway can turn almost any sandwich into a salad you'll love! Use the chart below to navigate your options based on your macros. (Be sure to add up the macros from each of the three categories.)

Salad Options:

Tuna salad (24g F | 15g P | 7g NC)

Veggie Delite (1g F | 3g P | 7g NC)

Chicken salad (4.5g F | 23g P | 8g NC)

Turkey breast (2g F | 12g P | 9g NC)

Toppings:

Black olives (3g F | 0g P | 0g NC)

Pickles (0g F | 0g P | 0g NC)

Jalapeños (0g F | 0g P | 0g NC)

Guacamole (6g F | 1g P | 1g NC)

Cucumbers (0g F | 0g P | 1g NC)

Tomatoes (0g F | 0g P | 1g NC)

Banana peppers (0g F | 0g P | 2g NC)

Dressings:

Chipotle Southwest (13g F | 0g P | 2g NC)

Oil and vinegar (7g F | 0g P | 0g NC)

Ranch (15g F | 0g P | 2g NC)

Caesar (18g F | 0g P | 2g NC)

Vinaigrette (7g F | 0g P | 2g NC)

Taco Bell

Taco Bell Power Bowls

Taco Bell Power Bowls are a great way to stay on track if you are on the go. Using the various toppings, you can mix and match to meet your macros. All of the options below are keto-friendly. Order by selecting your protein, toppings, and sauces.

Protein Base:

Beef (9g F | 10g P | 2g NC)

Chicken (3g F | 16g P | 0g NC)

Shredded chicken (7g F | 12g P | 2g NC)

Steak (4g F | 14g P | 2g NC)

Toppings:

Cheese (4g F | 3g P | 0g NC)

Bacon (5g F | 5g P | 0g NC)

Lettuce (0g F | 0g P | 0g NC)

Jalapeños (0g F | 0g P | 1g NC)

Onions (0g F | 0g P | 1g NC)

Pico de gallo (0g F | 0g P | 1g NC)

Guacamole (3g F | 0g P | 1g NC)

Sour cream (1.5g F | 0g P | 2g NC)

Tomatoes (0g F | 0g P | 0g NC)

Sauces:

Avocado Ranch (3.5g F | 3g P | 0g NC)

Creamy Chipotle (3g F | 0g P | 0g NC)

Spicy Ranch (3g F | 0g P | 0g NC)

Creamy Jalapeño (3g F | 0g P | 0g NC)

Green Chile Sauce (0g F | 0g P | 1g NC)

Mexican Pizza Sauce (0g F | 0g P | 2g NC)

Nacho Cheese Sauce (0g F | 0g P | 2g NC)

Red Sauce (0g F | 0g P | 2g NC)

Wendy's

Bunless Son of Baconator

Order a Son of Baconator with no bun and no ketchup.

37g F | 29g P | 4g NC (sandwich only)

Dave's Single Cheeseburger

Order a Dave's single cheeseburger with no ketchup and no bun.

29g F | 27g P | 3g NC (sandwich only)

Mexican Restaurants

Mexican food is a great option for your high-fat, low-carb lifestyle! Below you will find a list of best options and foods to avoid.

Fajitas

In general, fajitas are one of the best options at a Mexican food restaurant. I eat the meat, light onions (onions have carbs), sour cream, cheese, and guacamole.

Note: When you order, be sure to request no rice and beans. You can always replace the sides with sautéed vegetables or a side salad without croutons.

Entrée Salads

Entrée salads are another great option, but be sure to avoid corn, beans, croutons, taco shells, and tortilla chips. For dressing, ranch or Caesar are great choices.

Things to Avoid:

- Chips
- Tortillas
- Rice
- Beans
- Corn

Sushi Restaurants

There are several great low-carb options to choose from when dining at sushi restaurants.

Sashimi

These raw cuts of fish are great for keeping your carb count low. Be sure to skip the rice! Adding sliced avocado to sashimi can help increase the fats in this meal.

Riceless Rolls

Many sushi restaurants now offer a riceless roll selection. Don't see it on the menu? Ask the chef if there are any rolls that can be made without rice.

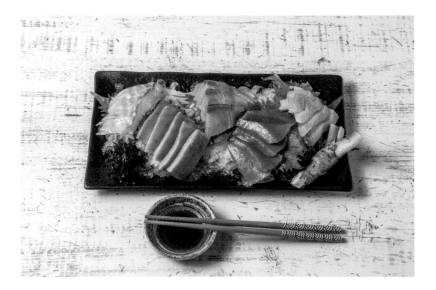

Steak Houses

When visiting a steak house, the typical menu involves a cut of meat and a variety of sides. Below are the best options when visiting a steak house.

Be sure to skip the bread that is often served. A Caesar salad is a great way to start the meal.

Main Courses

In general, all meats are great for our plan, but be sure the meat was not marinated in a sweet marinade. Fattier cuts of meat are best as meat is already so high in protein.

Side Dishes

Sautéed spinach	Asparagus	Side salad
Creamed spinach	Broccoli	Brussels sprouts

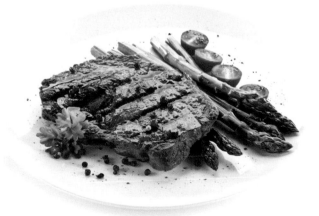

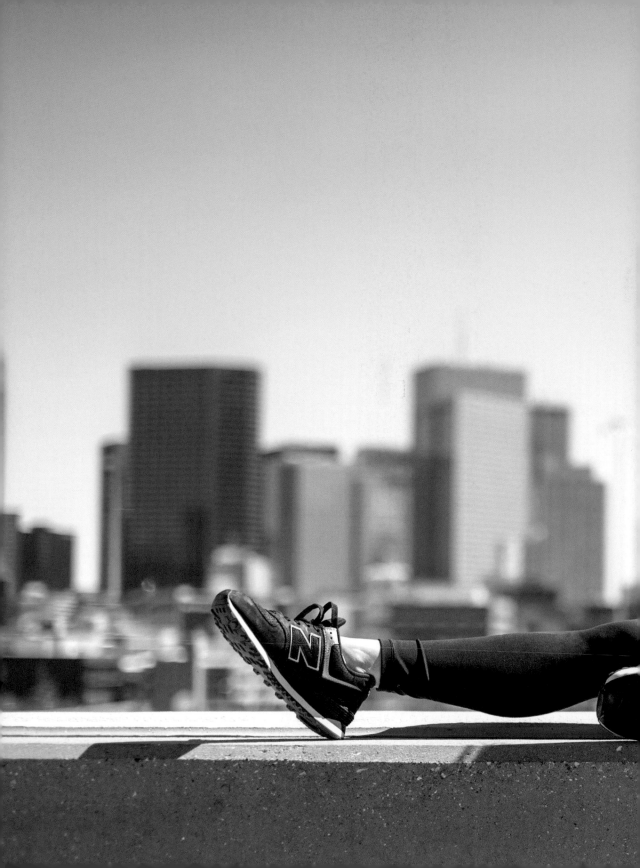

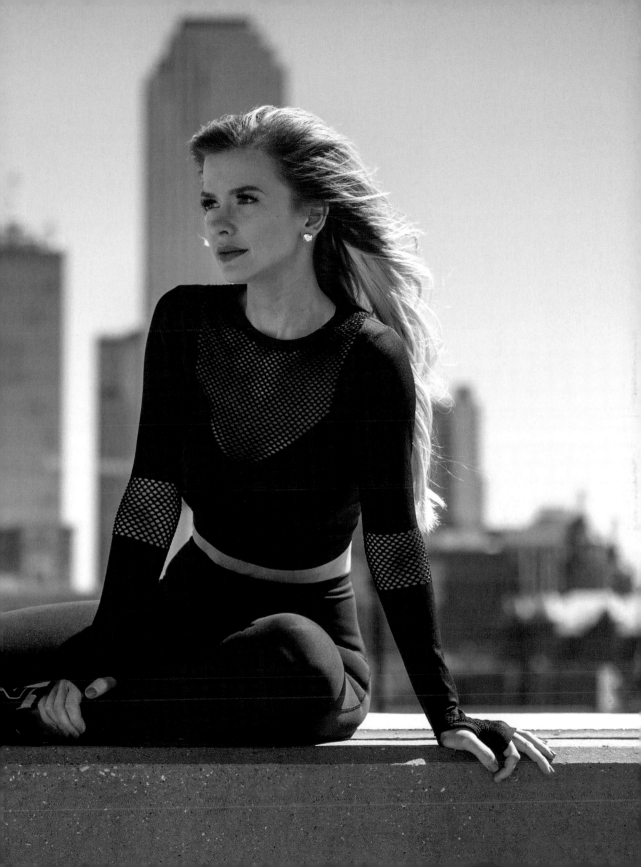

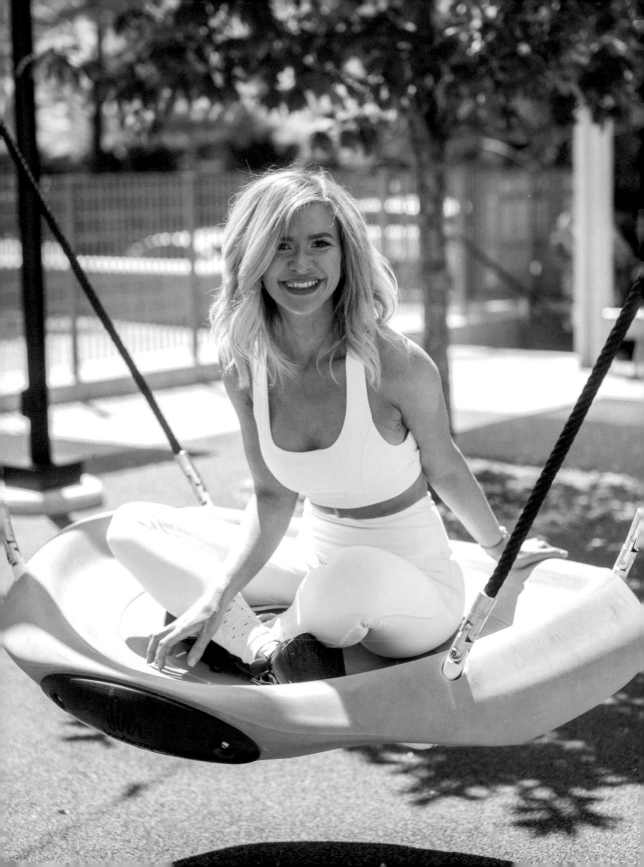

TAKE THE LEAP!

Well, here we are at the very end of our time together. We've learned a lot! I hope the things we covered have felt like a warm hug while also challenging you to become the best version of yourself. While we've reached the end of this book, you should consider it the introductory chapter to your new life and the story *you* are going to tell.

I hope you have already started working through some of the mindset exercises and have put a plan into place. If you haven't, that's okay! It's normal to feel a little apprehensive at first. Regardless of where you are at this moment, I want to encourage you to have the faith to start. Take a deep breath in, breathe out, and begin.

Fear can begin to get to us when we start something new. We know what we need to do, but the fear of change can feel terrifying. It's one thing to want your circumstances to change, and a whole different thing to realize *you* are the only one who has the power to change them.

This is your moment to change your life. You have a heroic story to tell, and it starts now. The dark moments of your life will no longer feel as

This is your moment to change your life.

though they have been in vain, because you are about to write a powerful story about how you overcame the giants you thought would crush you. You already have what it takes to win the war with food and begin a beautiful life you are proud of.

Just remember, the first step is always the hardest. Taking the leap is always a risk, but the risk is worth the reward. On days you struggle, lean into the mind-set chapters. On days you fall off track, pour over the recipes and pick a new one to try.

I promise you are far stronger than you realize, and I know you have the power inside of your heart to win this battle and make these changes. I believe in you!

NOTES

Chapter 1: Where It All Began

1. "Binge Eating Disorder," National Eating Disorders Association, https://www.nationaleatingdisorders.org/learn/by-eating-disorder/bed
2. Olivia Ryan, "Happiness Hormones: How They Differ and Why It Is Important," Thrive Global, March 30, 2018, https://thriveglobal.com/stories/happiness-hormones-how-they-differ-and-why-it-is-important/.

Chapter 5: Approaching a Keto Lifestyle

1. "How Much Sugar Do You Eat? You May Be Surprised," NH DHHS-DPHS Health Promotion in Motion, https://www.dhhs.nh.gov/dphs/nhp/documents/sugar.pdf.
2. "Frequently Asked Questions About Sugar," American Heart Association, July 27, 2018, https://www.heart.org/HEARTORG/HealthyLiving/HealthyEating/Nutrition/Frequently-Asked-Questions-About-Sugar_UCM_306725_Article.jsp.
3. "What Should Your Ketone Levels Be?," Keto-Mojo, https://keto-mojo.com/pages/what-should-your-ketone-levels-be.

Chapter 6: The Ketogenic Plan

1. Kris Gunnars, "Is Dairy Bad for You, or Good? The Milky, Cheesy Truth," Healthline, November 15, 2018, https://www.healthline.com/nutrition/is-dairy-bad-or-good#intolerance.

CREDITS

PHOTOGRAPHY
Leslee Mitchell Photography

MAKEUP & HAIR
Jenny Connors

PHOTOS BY LESLEE MITCHELL PHOTOGRAPHY
Cover, xii, 53, 54-55, 56, 72, 126, 132-133, 134, 141, and 146

ADDITIONAL PHOTOS BY DOMINGO RIVERA
iv, xxii, 1, 2, 5, 8, 13, 14, 16, 20, 26, 44, 75, 154-155, 156, 162, 176, 180, 181, 182, 184, 186, 187, 188, 189, 190, 191, 192, 193, 194, 195, 196, 197, 198, 199, 204, 205, 206, 208, 210, 211, 214, 215, 216, 217, 214, 218, 220, 242-243, 244

ADDITIONAL PHOTO CREDITS

ABOUT THE AUTHOR

Christine Carter is the founder and CEO of Weightlosshero LLC based in Texas. She is a Certified Fitness Trainer through AFAA and has a specialization in Behavior Change through NASM. Through her business she coaches those looking to sustain a healthier lifestyle and weight, encourages her large social media following daily, and she teaches and inspires people around the world via her YouTube channel.

· · · · · · · · · ·

Heather Rushin is a recipe developer and food photographer based in Seattle, Washington. Heather began developing nut-free ketogenic recipes and eventually began sharing them on her real food–based website, ARealFoodJourney.com. She most recently coauthored *Keto Clarity Cookbook* with keto expert Jimmy Moore.